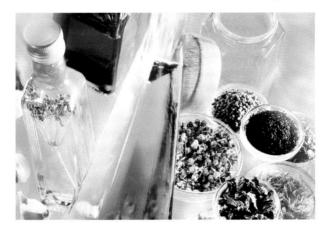

TANJA HIRSCHSTEINER

Home Remedies from A to Z

The Best Home and Natural Remedies

BARRON'S

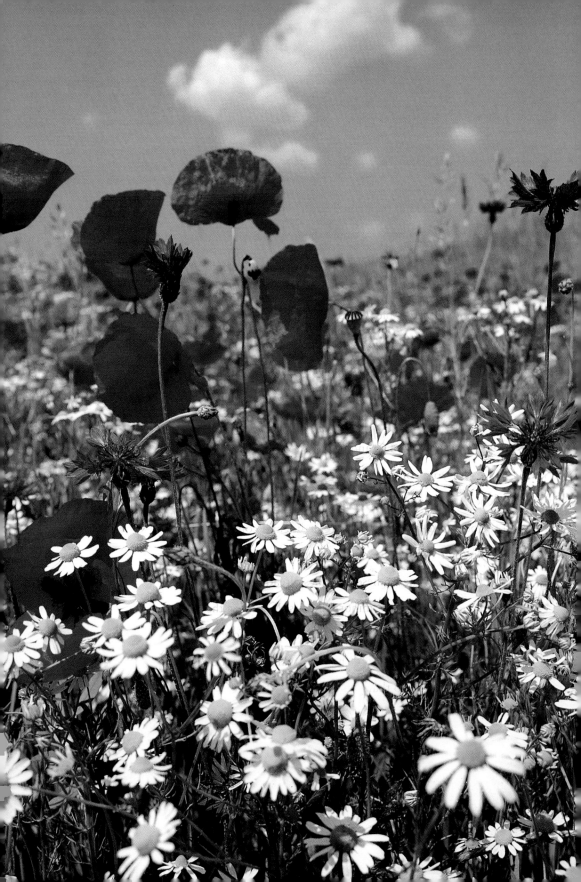

Preface

Did you know that honey can fight off almost any kind of bacteria? That pop singer Madonna drinks kombucha every morning? Why a glass of wine with dinner is better for you than drinking no alcohol at all? Have you always wanted to know what herbs can really do and how to use them correctly? Do you know when to use a cold pack, or when a warm wrap is called for?

If so, you are among the people who don't wish to check responsibility for their health at the door to the doctor's office. Prescription drugs and a surgeon's scalpel are reasonable and necessary in many cases. But there are many other, more gentle ways to prevent and treat illnesses!

In this book, I have compiled Grandmother's "secret remedies" and health tips for you, compared them with the latest findings of modern science, and brought them up-to-date. The result is a collection of the best tried-and-true home remedies and common herbs. I have provided information on their various uses and instructions on how to prepare them. You almost certainly have some of these remedies already in your home, so you can start using them immediately to treat minor ailments. If you use these natural "healing aides" regularly, you can stop many health problems before they start. I hope that this book will whet your appetite for honey, sauerkraut, garlic, spices, vegetable oils, green tea, and much more so that you won't get sick in the first place.

Tanja Hirschsteiner

Contents

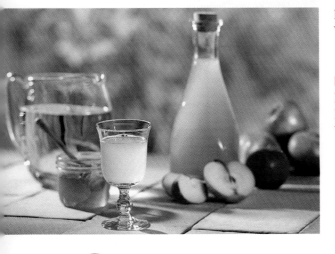

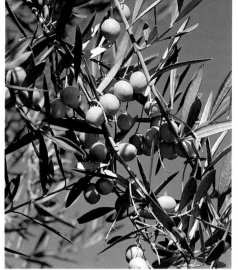

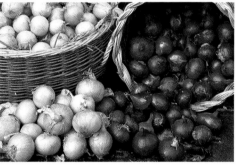

Contents

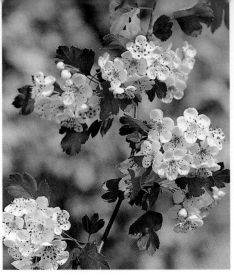

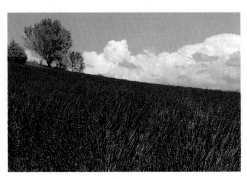

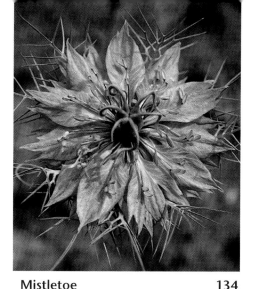

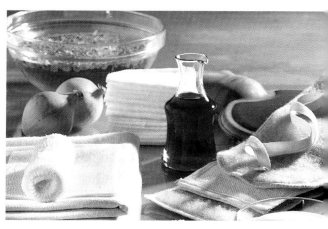

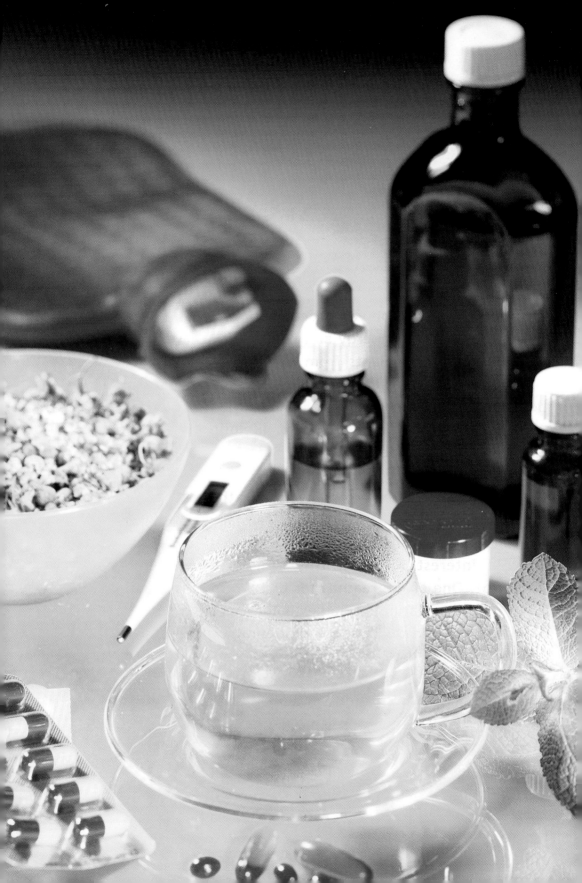

Nature's Gentle Aid

For thousands of years people have been turning to nature as a source of energy and health. They have been collecting herbs, using plants from their vegetable gardens as remedies, and utilizing the healing powers of water. Thanks to these natural treatments there have always been people who enjoy excellent lifelong health and live to a ripe, old age.

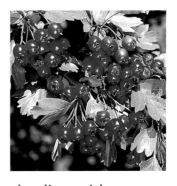

After a time when rapid advances in the fields of medicine and chemistry caused many people to lose faith in natural healing, there is renewed interest in using this time-tried knowledge. One of the reasons for this return to healing with herbs and other natural remedies is the fact that these treatments entail fewer dangers from undesirable side effects than modern medicine. Natural healing, however, should go hand in hand with proper nutrition and a healthy lifestyle. In fact, for any healing to occur body and soul must be in harmony; that, in fact, is something that natural remedies are known to promote.

Rediscovering the Tried-and-True

Of Priests, Nuns, and Grandmothers

A wealth of empirical knowledge was accumulated over many centuries

Long before medical knowledge was systematically compiled and recorded, it was primarily old women and village healers who collected a wealth of practical knowledge on how to treat many illnesses with plants, minerals, and other substances found in nature. This empirical knowledge grew and evolved in the monasteries and convents during the Middle Ages. Monks and nuns compared folk remedies with information on healing in ancient Greek and Roman texts, refined the methods through trial and error, and wrote down their findings. Saint Hildegard of Bingen, a nun who lived in the twelfth century, was perhaps the best known practitioner of this monastic medicine.

In the nineteenth century Samuel Hahnemann developed homeopathy, and J. S. Hahn and C. W. Hufeland advocated the use of hydrotherapy, a treatment that was later expanded by Sebastian Kneipp, a catholic priest. Kneipp prescribed cold water applications (affusions, washings, baths, treading water, packs, and compresses), as well as herbal preparations and a healthy lifestyle.

Our grandmothers knew the healing powers of nature and treated the entire family with such simple but effective remedies as herbal teas, juices, inhalations, and compresses. Natural remedies were passed down from generation to generation until, for several decades, they were nearly forgotten due to our blind faith in the progress of conventional modern medicine.

Healing Rituals

A patient needs attention

In order for patients to get well, their self-healing powers must be activated. This is accomplished by strengthening their immune system, and by enhancing their emotional and spiritual health. In their infirmaries, the monks and nuns of the Middle Ages prescribed the appropriate prayer along with a certain medicine. In the period before the Enlightenment, mythical faith and rituals were included in the treatment of the ill, a practice that greatly influenced their healing. In the typical medical practice of today, most patients receive little personal attention. Too often, only a few words are exchanged before the doctor gets out the prescription pad. Natural healing practices, in contrast, require a certain amount of time and involvement, a sort of ritual act. Even the simple task of preparing a cup of tea can be viewed as such an act. Treatments that require more time, such as administering a pack, provide a good opportunity to lovingly nurture the patient.

Getting Healthy, Staying Healthy

The purpose of this book is to help you use natural remedies correctly and to make you feel good about the different substances and treatments used in natural healing. There is much satisfaction in being able to contribute to and participate in one's own healing—or in helping others improve their health.

If you have little or no experience with home remedies and herbs, start with some simple remedies. Next time you have a headache, for example, drink a glass of cold water with two tablespoons of apple cider vinegar and a tablespoon of honey. It will work faster than your headache medicine, taste better—and it is guaranteed to have no side effects.

Try natural remedies for many other minor ailments as well. Women don't have to live with premenstrual syndrome, the discomfort commonly experienced before their period; chaste tree can help. The onset of decreased heart function, a condition that eventually affects everyone, and other age-related symptoms can be significantly delayed with hawthorn and a number of other herbs and home remedies. Garlic can lower slightly elevated blood pressure when synthetic medications can't be justified because of their side effects. St. John's wort is an effective remedy for seasonal affective disorder (SAD), a form of depression that commonly occurs in winter when sunshine is scarce. Most people find that this remedy quickly lifts their spirits and helps them find renewed energy and optimism.

Many ailments can be treated with natural remedies

Washings and affusions, healing herbs, and a healthy diet strengthen the body's immune system before infections can take hold that might later require treatment with antibiotics. And should you still get a cold after all, listen to your body's signals: what it's asking for is rest and loving attention.

Some Patience Is Required

Natural remedies won't necessarily make your aches and pains disappear as fast as you're accustomed to. A little patience and

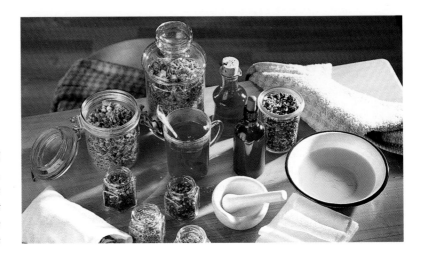

Dried herbs and tinctures for teas, baths, and packs should be part of your home health supplies

persistence, active cooperation, and sometimes discipline on the part of the patient are all part of the natural healing process. When disease has interfered with an organism for some time, it will take a while for the body to regain its equilibrium, and for health and well-being to return.

For a long-lasting recovery, certain life style changes are often necessary. Stress, in particular, must be reduced. Many people have to change their diet and get more exercise. These kinds of changes usually don't take place overnight.

 T!p

Expand Your First Aid Kit
Along with such standard items as a thermometer and pills for headaches, include some herbs for teas, baths, and inhaling, the materials for applying packs and compresses, and an aromatic body oil in your first aid kit. Everything you need for using these gentle natural remedies can be purchased at your pharmacy, health food store, or medical supply store; or you may already have it in your kitchen.

Important! *Important:* Always buy quality products so you can be sure that they contain an abundance of active ingredients.

It was Hippocrates by the way, whose oath every physician is required to take, who first advised that "Your foods should be medicines and your medicines should be foods." His concept of healing was based on a structured lifestyle, sound nutrition, and herbal remedies.

Limitations of Self-treatment

Minor complaints without any serious underlying cause are the kinds of ailments you can safely treat yourself. However, if the symptoms are not specific or are hard to describe, or if they do not improve within three days, you should always consult a doctor or other health care practitioner. With his or her agreement you may be able to combine standard medical treatment with natural remedies, which may shorten the course of the illness. The treatment of serious diseases with natural remedies and healing practices should only be done by a qualified, experienced practitioner.

Even herbs aren't always perfectly harmless or free from unwanted side effects. Watch out for allergic reactions or other signs of intolerance.

Always remember: A proper diagnosis is necessary before any treatment

What This Book Can Do for You

In the first part of this book you will find descriptions of the most important remedies from your kitchen, such as the versatile apple cider vinegar or the onion. Although they are mainly used to promote health and prevent illness, these remedies can also complement conventional treatment for certain ailments. For many minor complaints these natural remedies can bring quick relief without side effects.

In the second chapter, you become familiar with the most popular herbs. You will find out how to use them and how they work. You will also learn about some tried-and-true herbal tea mixtures.

All the various water applications—baths, affusions, washings, packs, compresses—are described in the chapter on hydrotherapy. Here you will find detailed instructions on how and when to use these remedies for best results.

An extensive chart of ailments at the end of the book refers you straight to the specific chapters where they are discussed. For instance, if you are suffering from poor blood circulation, you can see at a glance what remedies are appropriate for your condition and the specific chapter and page where you can find them.

Relieve your aches and pains with remedies found in your kitchen, your herb garden, and from your water faucet

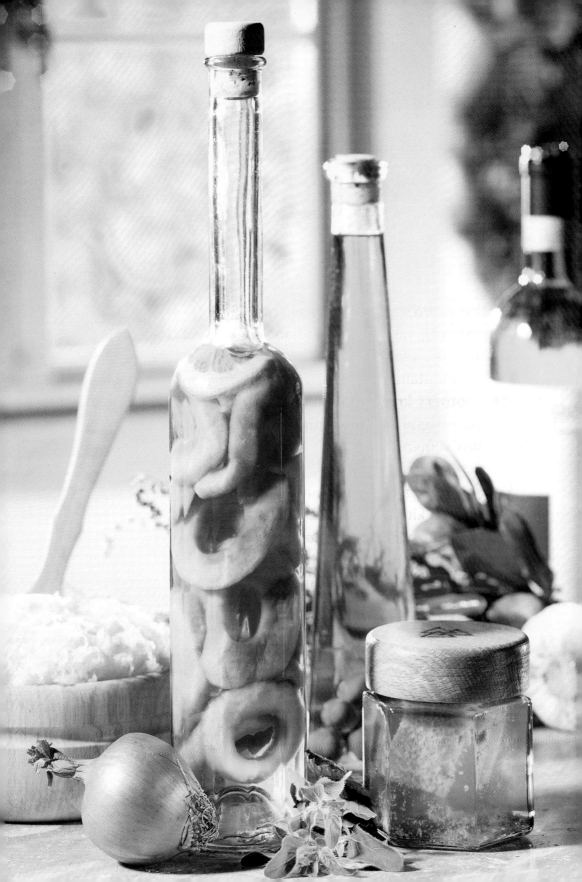

Remedies from Your Kitchen

All the world's major medical traditions, from medieval European monastic medicine to Indian Ayurveda, to traditional Chinese medicine, teach that proper nutrition plays as important a role in maintaining and restoring health as do medicines. Our grandmothers knew that many common foods are very useful for preventing and even curing various ailments.

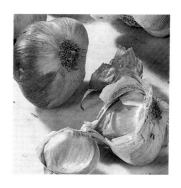

You probably already have more natural remedies in your kitchen than you realize. In this chapter you will learn how you can improve your general health with apple cider vinegar, spices, honey, kefir, common culinary herbs, vegetable oils, sauerkraut, and other foods, and how they can be used to treat many ailments. As is the case with medications, the correct dosage and manner of preparation are often crucial for success. All the recipes contained in this book are easy to prepare and use. With a little practice, treating yourself and your family with natural, effective and inexpensive remedies from your kitchen will become second nature to you.

Apple Cider Vinegar

A Fountain of Youth Offering Health and Beauty

Vinegar in all sorts of varieties has been used for thousands of years, not only for seasoning but also as a beverage, a natural medicine, and a preservative. As far back as 3000 B.C. vinegar was produced in breweries along with beer. During the Middle Ages vinegar was enriched with berries, flowers, and herbs, and it was subject to taxation. Hildegard of Bingen mentioned the beneficial effects of vinegar on digestion. For many centuries vinegar was indispensable for hygiene: long before bacteria were discovered to be the cause of disease, wounds were cleaned and sick rooms disinfected with vinegar. The smelling salts used by the ladies of the upper classes contained aromatic vinegar.

How Apple Cider Vinegar is Made

Vinegar is produced when acetic acid bacteria act on alcoholic liquids in the presence of oxygen. This happens whenever an alcoholic substance is left standing. Vinegar, therefore, didn't need to be invented. It only had to be discovered, and it still is a natural product today. Making apple cider vinegar is simple: apples are pressed and the juice is allowed to ferment. The resulting alcohol is turned into acetic acid by bacteria. Since apple wine contains less alcohol than grape wine, the resulting apple cider vinegar is less acidic than wine vinegar. Apple cider vinegar tastes fruity and only mildly sour.

Acetic acid itself contains no valuable substances. Its only useful property is that it removes stubborn dirt and stains

How Apple Cider Vinegar Works

Apple cider vinegar contains minerals and trace elements such as calcium, fluoride, magnesium, sodium, phosphorus, and silicon. It is also very rich in potassium, which is important for the heart muscle. Another active ingredient is pectin, a type of dietary fiber with cholesterol-lowering properties that is present in substantial amounts especially in unfiltered apple cider vinegar. In addition to water and acetic acid, apple cider vinegar contains some residual alcohol and various by-products of fermentation. All in all, it is a very complex liquid whose regenerative and healing properties are the result of the synergy of all its active ingredients.

Its most important effect is antibacterial and mostly due to the presence of acetic acid. At a specific concentration, this acid destroys its own bacteria. This limits the acid level of naturally produced vinegar to a certain maximum.

The antibacterial properties of apple cider vinegar have a beneficial effect on the digestive tract. They aid the natural bacteria required for proper digestion, the intestinal flora, by killing harmful bacteria that cause decay and unhealthy fermentation. Apple cider vinegar also improves digestion and helps maintain a healthy ratio of acids to bases in the body. This balance can be upset by stress, chronic illness, or by eating processed foods. The result is too much acid throughout the organism. Excessive acidity can be counteracted by vegetables, fruit, and other unprocessed foods that act as bases. Although they taste acidic, apple cider vinegar and lemons belong in this category of foods, since they act as bases inside the body.

In the respiratory pathways the vapors of apple cider vinegar destroy germs, increase blood circulation, and reduce bronchial mucus. Studies have shown that people involved in the production of vinegar who regularly inhale its vapors have significantly fewer respiratory infections.

How exactly apple cider vinegar works and which substances are responsible for its specific benefits are not yet known.

How to Use Apple Cider Vinegar

When buying apple cider vinegar, insist on good quality: Choose only naturally fermented vinegar. The apples used should preferably be organic, since peel and core, the parts most likely to contain pesticides, are usually not removed from fruits used for vinegar production.

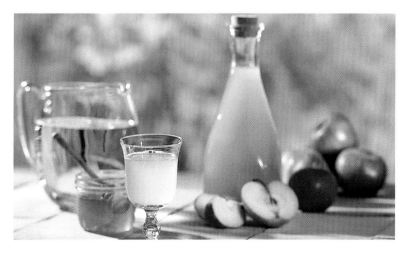

Apple cider vinegar diluted with water and sweetened with honey tastes good and is an effective treatment for many ailments

Apple Cider Vinegar-Honey Drink

▶ Apple cider vinegar and honey are two home remedies that complement each other exceptionally well. Add 2 tablespoons of apple cider vinegar and 1 tablespoon of honey to 1 glass of water and stir well. Drink in small sips. With an apple cider vinegar cure, which should last for about six weeks, drink two to three glasses of the mixture every day.

Inhaling

▶ Pour a half-pint of apple cider vinegar into a bowl and add about half a quart of hot water. Lean over the bowl and drape a hand towel like a tent over your head and the bowl. Inhale the rising steam for five to ten minutes.

Baths, Compresses, and Washings with Apple Cider Vinegar

These applications are described in detail on pages 157, 163, and 169.

When to Use Apple Cider Vinegar

Apple cider vinegar has a revitalizing effect on the entire organism. It stimulates the body's metabolism and also provides a significant amount of the daily requirements of minerals and vitamins. It acts as a digestive aid and inhibits the spread of bacteria in the body. Although it is first and foremost a wholesome food that helps the body stay healthy, it can also be used to treat minor ailments.

Restoring General Health, Purification, and Prevention

An apple cider vinegar cure—for instance in the spring and the fall—revitalizes the entire body after a long winter, a prolonged illness, or chronic exhaustion. By adjusting the intestinal flora it aids in digestion and strengthens the immune system. Apple cider vinegar can further be used along with regular medical treatment for chronic headaches, circulatory problems, and cardiovascular weakness. It also inhibits the formation of kidney and gallstones. If you would like to lose a few pounds in the course of a spring cure, you should also drink apple cider vinegar every day.

Main Applications at a Glance

Ailments:	Suggested Applications:
Abdominal gas	Apple cider vinegar drink
Acne	Steam bath for the face; drink
Bruises, sprains, strains	Cold or warm packs
Cardiovascular problems	Washings; cold packs; drink
Colds	Inhaling; drink
Constipation	Warm stomach packs, drink
Cough, bronchitis	Inhaling; cold or warm chest packs; drink
Detoxification	Treatment with apple cider vinegar drink
Diarrhea	Drink diluted apple cider vinegar
Headaches	Drink; cold compress on the forehead
Hemorrhoids	Sitz baths
Immune deficiency	Apple cider vinegar cure, washings
Insect stings	Cold packs or compresses
Menstrual problems	Apple cider vinegar-honey drink
Nausea	Apple cider vinegar-honey drink
Overweight	Apple cider vinegar-honey drink cure
Rheumatoid conditions	Drink; cold or warm packs
Skin rash	Apply and rub in apple cider vinegar; drink
Sore throat	Inhaling; moist, hot throat packs; drink
Sunburn	Compresses; lukewarm bath
Urinary bladder infection	Apple cider vinegar drink
Vaginal discharge	Douches; drink
Varicose veins	Cold leg packs; foot baths; washings

Recipes

▶ *Immune deficiency:*
Take an apple cider vinegar cure, along with regular washings with apple cider vinegar (see page 169).
Apple cider vinegar cure: Drink two to three glasses of apple cider vinegar and honey daily for about six weeks. If you would like to lose weight, add only a small amount of honey.
▶ *Chronic headaches:*
For chronic headaches, do an apple cider vinegar cure and apply cold compresses to the forehead (see 161).
▶ *Cardiovascular problems:*
Do an apple cider vinegar cure. Do regular washings and in the morning apply cold wraps to your calves with apple cider vinegar (see pages 157 and 168).

Infections

Apple cider vinegar is also useful as an adjunct treatment for colds, upper respiratory infections and cystitis (urinary bladder infections). Adding honey to the vinegar enhances its antibacterial action and provides additional active ingredients.

Recipes

▶ *Urinary bladder infection:*
Drinking lots of fluids is the most important factor in treating bladder infections. You should drink three quarts of fluids daily to flush out harmful bacteria. Alternate between a cup of herbal bladder tea and a glass of apple cider vinegar-honey drink.
▶ *Bronchitis, coughs, colds:*
Inhale twice daily with apple cider vinegar and apply chest wraps (warm ones for chronic conditions, cold ones for acute ailments; see page 159). In addition, drink three glasses of apple cider vinegar-honey drink a day.
▶ *Sore throat:*
As soon as you notice the first scratching sensation, gargle as often as possible with a mixture of two tablespoons of water and one tablespoon of apple cider vinegar. Drink three glasses of apple cider vinegar-honey drink every day and apply moist-hot wraps to the throat twice a day (see page 158).

Sports Injuries and Rheumatoid Conditions

A mixture of mineral water, apple cider vinegar, and honey makes an ideal thirst-quencher after all kinds of sports activities. It contains the right amounts of all the important minerals that are lost during exercise, thereby preventing mineral deficiencies that could lead to muscle cramps.

Various sports injuries can be easily treated with apple cider vinegar. Taken regularly, it reduces swelling, alleviates joint pain due to arthritic or rheumatoid conditions, and reduces stiffness in the joints for many people.

▶ *Sports drink:*
Add two tablespoons of apple cider vinegar and one tablespoon of honey to a large glass of mineral water.

▶ *Joint pains, rheumatoid conditions:*
Drink two glasses of apple cider vinegar and honey every day for an extended period. Increase the amount for acute conditions. Treat acute joint inflammation with a cold wrap applied to the affected area every day. For chronic conditions apply at least one warm wrap per week. Get plenty of exercise to prevent stiffening of the joints.

▶ *Bruises:*
Apply a cold wrap with apple cider vinegar immediately to reduce swelling (see page 157). Repeat as needed.

▶ *Strains and sprains:*
Sports injuries that respond to heat can be treated with a moist-hot wrap (see page 158) with apple cider vinegar.

Recipes

Women's Ailments

Some of the minerals contained in apple cider vinegar, such as potassium, calcium, and magnesium, play an important part in muscle metabolism and pain relief. That's why apple cider vinegar is an effective treatment for menstrual cramps caused by painful contractions of the uterine muscles. Regular intake of apple cider vinegar can help provide some of the minerals the body requires in increased amounts during pregnancy. It can also alleviate nausea commonly experienced during the first trimester.

When used externally, apple cider vinegar can also prevent vaginal infections. Added to vaginal douches, it relieves minor itching or burning of the vaginal mucous membranes.

Important: If symptoms persist for several days, you must see a gynecologist. There could be a serious condition requiring diagnosis and treatment.

+ See a doctor

▶ *Menstrual pain:*
Drink at least one glass of apple cider vinegar-honey drink regularly.

▶ *Morning sickness during pregnancy:*
Drink a glass of apple cider vinegar-honey drink first thing in the morning.

Recipes

▶ *Vaginal Yeast Infection:*
Use a vaginal douche of equal parts apple cider vinegar and luke-warm water twice a day. You can use a large plastic syringe (available at your pharmacy).

Weak Veins

This is a condition where blood flow is impaired because the walls of the veins have lost their normal tone and elasticity. The result is varicose veins. Due to its astringent and anti-inflammatory properties, apple cider vinegar is effective in treating heavy, swollen legs, varicose veins, and even hemorrhoids.

Recipes

▶ *Varicose Veins, Swollen Legs:*
Apply cold leg wraps (see page 160), or use regular cold foot baths (page 164) or washings (page 168) with apple cider vinegar, especially when you experience acute symptoms.

▶ *Hemorrhoids:*

Constipation and straining during bowel movements can aggravate hemorrhoids

If you frequently suffer from painful hemorrhoids, take regular sitz baths with lukewarm water and apple cider vinegar or dried chamomile (see page 163). For acute symptoms, you can apply a piece of cotton saturated with apple cider vinegar to reduce swelling and relieve pain.

Digestive Ailments

Apple cider vinegar promotes a healthy intestinal flora. This makes it an effective and fast-acting remedy for abdominal gas, stomach pains, feeling of fullness, nausea, and abdominal cramps due to sluggish digestion. If symptoms persist or keep recurring, a cure with apple cider vinegar (see page 18) may help. In the case of diarrhea, apple cider vinegar works as an antibacterial agent, and at the same time it replenishes the minerals your body has lost. Do not add honey in this case, however, because it has a slight tendency to cause diarrhea.

Important!

Important: Make sure your doctor rules out such chronic intestinal disorders as Crohn's disease or colitis ulcerosa as a possible cause of your symptoms!

Recipes

▶ *Abdominal Gas, Feeling of Fullness, Nausea:*
Drink a glass of apple cider vinegar-honey drink before each meal.

▶ *Diarrhea:*
Drink a mixture of two tablespoons of apple cider vinegar and a glass of mineral water several times a day.

▶ *Constipation:*
Drink several glasses of lukewarm apple cider vinegar-honey drink every day. Warm abdominal wraps with apple cider vinegar (see page 160) can also help.

Skin and Hair Problems

Apple cider vinegar is also beneficial when applied externally. It improves blood circulation to the skin, helps clear up rashes due to allergies, relieves itching, and reduces swelling from bug bites. Good blood circulation to the skin facilitates removal of metabolic by-products and environmental toxins from the body. As a result, the skin looks healthier, and acne visibly improves. Diluted apple cider vinegar cools minor burns including sunburn, relieves pain, and helps prevent scars. Applied regularly, it leaves the skin more supple and gives it a healthy glow. Hair, too, becomes softer, shinier, and easier to comb. Regular rinsing with apple cider vinegar is even said to delay the onset of graying.

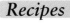

Recipes

▶ *Allergic Rashes:*
Mix equal parts of apple cider vinegar and cold water, add a little honey, and rub the mixture into the affected area several times a day. For best results, saturate a piece of cotton with the mixture, place it on the affected area, and secure it with adhesive tape.

▶ *Insect Bites:*
Apply a cold apple cider vinegar wrap to the swollen area. For minor stings, dip a small cloth or gauze in diluted apple cider vinegar, squeeze out any excess liquid, and place it on the affected area.

▶ *Acne:*
Twice a week, use a facial steam bath (see *Inhaling*, page 18), followed by rinsing with a mixture of equal parts of apple cider vinegar and cold water to close the pores.

▶ *Mild Sunburn:*
Cool the sunburned area repeatedly with apple cider vinegar compresses (see page 162). A lukewarm bath, with a half-pint of apple cider vinegar added to the water, also relieves burning.

▶ *Brittle, Over-Processed Hair:*
Mix one part apple cider vinegar with one part warm water and apply to washed hair while still wet. Leave in for a few minutes, then rinse thoroughly.

Garlic

Warding Off Demons and Diseases

Garlic is one of the oldest medicinal plants known to man. It is first mentioned as a remedy and a spice in ancient Sumerian texts written almost 5000 years ago. Later, Greeks, Romans, and various Germanic tribes used garlic for the same purposes. In Europe, the plant has been widely known since the Middle Ages, when Benedictine monks grew it in the gardens of their monasteries and used it to protect people from infectious epidemics. During the years when the plague ravaged Marseille, bands of thieves who robbed the sick and the dead claimed that the consumption of garlic pickled in wine and vinegar gave them immunity from the disease.

Garlic also performs another important function. For centuries, people have hung it in their doorways and windows to drive away demons, witches, and vampires.

Bulbils with seeds grow on the tall stems of the garlic plant

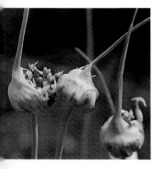

How to Identify Garlic

Garlic (*Allium sativum*) originated in the Orient, but it is widely cultivated in Europe, Africa, and the Americas. The plant prefers sunny locations and loose, sandy soil rich in nutrients. Tall stems, up to three feet high, grow from a main bulb consisting of several cloves. Its slender leaves resemble the leek, and it bears reddish-white flowers from June to August. The flower heads are later replaced by secondary bulbs that measure about a half-inch in diameter and contain seeds.

How to Plant and Harvest Garlic

A great way to dry garlic is to harvest the entire plant, tie the leaves of several plants together into a braid, and hang it up

Garlic grows best in heavy, well-fertilized soil. It prefers only moderate watering. You can propagate garlic by either using cloves or bulbils. Both are planted in March/April or September/October. Arrange them in rows, with the individual plants spaced about six inches apart, and about eight inches between rows. If you plant bulbils, it will take two years until you can harvest a crop. You can also grow garlic plants in clay pots on your deck or porch. Harvest the bulbs when the leafy tops have dried out in the fall. Most of the commercially produced garlic, often grown in large plantations, is processed into powder immediately after it's harvested.

What Makes Garlic So Effective

The main active ingredient of garlic is allicin. The amount contained in each bulb varies depending on where it was grown. Garlic cultivated in China is richest in allicin. Allicin is produced only when the cells of the fresh garlic bulb are crushed. Garlic also contains other active ingredients such as enzymes, amino acids, and hormone-like substances that function like male and female sex hormones.

Garlic dilates the blood vessels and acts as a blood thinner, thus improving cardiovascular function and lowering blood pressure. It has antioxidant properties, reduces excessive levels of cholesterol in the blood, and prevents cholesterol deposits in the arteries. All these actions reduce the risk of atherosclerosis. Garlic is an inexpensive alternative to cholesterol-lowering drugs for people with slightly high cholesterol levels.

A good alternative treatment for atherosclerosis

Garlic is also a sought-after remedy for its antibacterial properties. It is not quite as potent as antibiotics, but its effects are long lasting and it produces no undesirable side effects. Garlic can be used to combat some bacterial strains that have become resistant to antibiotics. By killing harmful bacteria and yeasts, it reduces undesirable fermentation in the intestine. Garlic stimulates bile production and it helps relieve painful abdominal cramps.

It is further said to inhibit the growth of tumors, lower blood sugar levels, and reduce the effects of various poisons.

Undesirable Side Effects

Garlic very rarely causes gastrointestinal complaints, allergic reactions, or cardiovascular problems. Some people can't tolerate large amounts of raw garlic and should avoid eating it on an empty stomach. People on medication for hypertension should consult their doctor before adding significant amounts of garlic to their diet.

How to Use Garlic

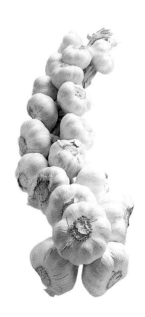

Garlic needs to be ingested over extended periods of time in order to be effective. The recommended daily dosage is at least $1/10$ ounce of fresh garlic (about 3 small cloves), 900 mg of garlic powder, or nine enteric-coated tablets.

Fresh Garlic

Fresh garlic can be added as a flavoring to many everyday foods.

Enteric-coated Tablets

Taking garlic in the form of enteric-coated tablets reduces undesirable odors

This form of supplement is appropriate for people who don't like to eat large amounts of raw garlic on a daily basis, or who want to make sure that they get enough garlic to enjoy its many health benefits. Enteric-coated tablets contain garlic powder obtained by a gentle drying process and are as effective as raw garlic.

Garlic Juice

Fresh garlic juice is easy to prepare.

Recipe

▶ *This is what you need:*
5 garlic cloves, 5 teaspoons of honey, water
▶ *This is how it's done:*
Crush or finely chop the garlic cloves. Mix in 5 teaspoons of honey. Add a half-pint of lukewarm water, steep for ten minutes, then strain through a cloth. Prepare fresh every day.

Soft Gelatin Capsules

Soft gelatin capsules sold in health food and natural food stores contain an oily extract. These preparations are not as effective as fresh garlic or garlic powder produced with minimal processing.

Fermented Garlic Products

The garlic in these products has been virtually "pre-digested" by chemical processes and is completely odorless. Along with the odor, these preparations probably have lost most of their health benefits.

Homeopathic Preparations

Homeopathic practitioners use garlic primarily to treat chronic bronchitis, digestive problems, rheumatic conditions, muscle and joint pain, and as a "garlic cure" for ailments associated with aging.

When to Use Garlic

Garlic is mainly used for its antibacterial and antifungal properties, and for its beneficial effects on cardiovascular function.

Main Applications at a Glance

Ailments:	Suggested Applications:
Bronchitis, cough	Drink garlic juice
Cardiovascular problems	Eat fresh garlic or take a garlic supplement
Diarrhea	Take garlic in high doses
Digestive problems	Eat fresh garlic or take a garlic supplement
Fungal skin infections or thrush	Dab with garlic juice; garlic compresses
Headaches	Eat fresh garlic or take a garlic supplement
Hypertension, elevated cholesterol	Eat fresh garlic or take a garlic supplement
To improve general health	Eat fresh garlic or take a garlic supplement
Unhealthy intestinal flora	Cure with fresh garlic or a garlic supplement

General Health

Garlic can improve your mood, increase physical stamina, and enhance your ability to concentrate. It reduces anxiety and has a calming effect on the nervous system.
▶ Take plenty of garlic, either fresh or in the form of a supplement, every day.

Recipe

Cardiovascular System

When taken regularly over several years, garlic can prevent, or at least reduce, changes in the blood vessels that could lead to strokes, kidney dysfunction, circulation problems in the legs, or reduced blood flow to the brain. People who suffer from headaches or tend to have cold hands and feet can also benefit from increased garlic intake. Consumed in sufficient amounts, garlic improves blood flow to all the organs and tissues, including the skin.

Recipe

✚ **See a doctor**

▶ Make sure that you get an adequate amount (1/10 ounce) of garlic every day. This will help prevent hardening of the arteries. If your cholesterol level is too high, avoid sugar and use only olive or canola oil. If you have elevated blood pressure, talk to your doctor before consuming extra garlic.

Digestive Ailments

The active ingredients found in garlic aid digestion and reduce fermentation in the intestines that could lead to abdominal gas, diarrhea, or painful cramps. Garlic can also relieve feelings of fullness, belching, and nausea.

Recipes

▶ *General indigestion:*
Consume 1/10 ounce of garlic every day.
▶ *Diarrhea:*
For acute conditions, ingest ten raw cloves of garlic or an equivalent amount of garlic supplements daily. Such a high dosage is necessary in order to achieve the desired effect.
▶ *Unhealthy intestinal flora:*
Follow a garlic cure of three to four weeks' duration. This is recommended particularly after a course of antibiotics.

Respiratory Ailments

In folk medicine, garlic is also used to treat ailments of the respiratory tract, such as bronchitis and coughs. It is also helpful in relieving the symptoms of whooping cough. However, whooping cough is a serious illness that always requires treatment by a doctor.

✚ **See a doctor**

Recipe

▶ Take spoonfuls of freshly squeezed garlic juice from five cloves in doses spread throughout the day.

Skin Infections

When minor wounds become infected, or when you are suffering from a fungal infection of the skin, try garlic for its antibacterial and antifungal properties. It often kills germs just as effectively as artificial preparations.

Recipes

▶ *Bacterial infections:*
Open a soft gelatin capsule and dab the affected area with garlic oil several times a day. As an alternative, you can apply compresses soaked in garlic oil (page 162).
▶ *Fungal infections:*
Dab the affected area with fresh garlic juice several times a day, or apply compresses soaked in garlic oil.

Green Tea

Miracle Cure from China

No one knows when people first made tea from the leaves of a plant. Legend has it that it was the Chinese emperor Shen Nung, also known as the "father of medicine," who discovered how to make tea by accident while on a hunting trip almost 5000 years ago. He was boiling water for drinking when a few leaves from a tea plant fell into his pot. The water took on a golden color and gave off a pleasant smell. When the emperor drank it, he was delighted with its taste and immediately felt refreshed and reinvigorated.

In China, tea plants were originally grown only for medicinal purposes in the gardens of monasteries. It took some time for tea to became popular as a reasonably priced alternative to fermented beverages among the general population.

From remedy to popular beverage

About 1000 years ago green tea was introduced to Tibet and Japan; in the 17th century it found its way via Russia to England, where the members of the aristocracy learned to enjoy it. By the middle of the 19th century fermented black tea grown on plantations in the British colonies had replaced green tea in Europe. Within the last few years, however, green tea has experienced a true renaissance because it's easy to digest and it entails various health benefits.

What the Tea Plant Looks Like

Both green and black tea are made from the leaves of the tea plant (*Camellia sinensis*, *Thea sinensis*), an evergreen tree that can grow to nearly fifty feet in height. Its dark green, serrated leaves are somewhat leathery, and it bears white or pink flowers that give off a pleasant scent.

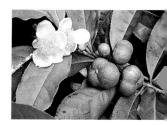

Flowers and fruits of the tea plant

An Overview of the Main Varieties

There are more than 150 varieties of green tea, among them some with artificial flavors that are generally avoided by true tea connoisseurs. For people who want to drink green tea for its medicinal properties, but who don't like its bitter taste, there are many high quality varieties that are flavored with natural fruit additives. Of course you can simply add some sugar or honey, or a small amount of lemon juice to the tea.

Variety	Characteristics	Color and Taste
Japan		
Bancha	similar to Sencha, rolled leaves slightly larger; classic variety, very popular	bright green color, fresh-tangy taste
Genmaicha	specialty made from Bancha and roasted whole brown rice	slightly brown color, slightly salty-grainy, sweetish taste
Gabalong	excellent quality; is regarded as health-promoting tea in Japan	very aromatic
Kokaicha	powdered, pressed leaves	bright yellow color, fresh, aromatic taste
Matcha	used in Japanese tea ceremonies; shrubs grow in the shade of deciduous trees; is briefly stirred with a bamboo whisk after brewing; relatively high in caffeine	bitter taste
Sencha	most popular tea in Japan; comes in three grades: superior, medium, and low	greenish-yellowish infusion; fragrant, fresh, light taste
China		
Green Pekoe	made from the bud and the first two leaves growing in spring; thin, carefully rolled leaves	bright green color, fresh taste
Gunpowder	leaves rolled into balls, open when infused; very high caffeine content	yellowish-green color, clear, fresh-bitter taste, very stimulating
Gu Zhang Mao Jian	only the most tender leaves are harvested ten days of the year; slightly fermented	especially light, slightly sweet taste
Ju Hua Cha	special delicacy: 50 young shoots are bound into a "tea rose"; opened in the cup and infused with hot water, it develops its great flavor	light yellow color, soft taste
Lung Ching	one of China's best teas; long, flat leaves	emerald green, light tea, soft, slightly sweet taste, pleasant, cooling effect
Oolong	very precious, because it's half fermented (innermost part of leaves is not fermented); between black and green tea	different tastes according to variety
Young Hyson	picked from wild tea plants; thick leaves are rolled into long, thin shape	full-bodied taste, stimulating, mild

Cultivating and Harvesting Green Tea

Every year, about 2.5 million tons of tea are produced world-wide. Twenty percent of that amount is green tea. Tea is grown mainly in South and East Asia, but also in South America, East Africa, the states of the former Soviet Union, Turkey, and Iran. Japan and China produce mostly green tea. Teas grown in India and Sri Lanka are typically black.

Tea plants grow best on higher elevations and in warm, humid climates. For ease in harvesting, it's grown in the shape of a shrub.

India alone produces 30 percent of the world's tea

The leaves, still picked largely by hand, are steamed, rolled, and dried immediately after harvesting. That way the enzymes don't change, and chemical content and color are preserved. In China, even green tea is usually slightly fermented and then roasted, which gives the brew, or infusion, a slightly orange hue. In contrast, brewed Japanese green tea is more greenish-yellow in color.

Unlike green tea, the leaves used to make black tea are slightly withered before they are rolled and then allowed to ferment under very humid conditions. This process, brought on by the enzymes contained in the leaves, turns them reddish-brown and then black, after drying. This process ensures that the caffeine contained in the tea can be quickly absorbed by the body, making the brew more stimulating. Unfortunately, some of its important active ingredients are also destroyed in the process, and the tea no longer serves as a remedy, but merely a as beverage.

What Makes Green Tea So Valuable

Perhaps the most impressive medicinal property of green tea stems from two of its chemical constituents, tannin and catechin, both very effective antioxidants surpassing even vitamin E. Antioxidants may slow down the aging process in the body, may inhibit the growth of cancerous cells, and protect the organism from the effects of harmful ultra-violet rays. Green tea is also very beneficial to the cardiovascular system because it reduces harmful deposits in the blood vessels (arteriosclerosis). In addition, it acts as an anticoagulant and lowers the levels of harmful lipids in the blood. The tea's enzymes can even lower slightly elevated blood pressure and thereby reduce the risk of heart attack and stroke. It may also aid cell function and regeneration throughout the entire body, is useful in treating metabolic disorders, such as diabetes and gout, and strengthens the immune system.

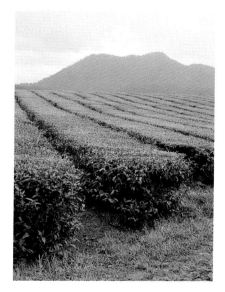

A typical tea plantation in India

Green tea's main
constituents are
tannin, caffeine,
catechins,
vitamins,
and minerals

The tannins in green tea stimulate appetite and aid digestion. They have an astringent effect on the mucous membranes of the intestinal tract, and therefore relieve diarrhea. Caffeine gets absorbed more slowly, so the tea's stimulting effect is milder and longer lasting than that of black tea.

Caffeine Is Beneficial to Your Health
Caffeine taken in proper doses stimulates the central nervous system as well as respiration, aids the function of the heart, and relieves headaches, migraines, and rheumatoid conditions. The small, young leaves of the green tea plant contain more caffeine than the older ones. People who have high blood pressure should choose green tea varieties with low caffeine content and generally avoid black tea.

Green tea is rich in minerals and trace minerals, and therefore is good for your teeth. Children who drink a cup of green tea a day or use it regularly as a mouthwash may reduce their risk of cavities. Green tea also contains zinc, a mineral needed especially during pregnancy, and high amounts of vitamin A, C, the B vitamins, and volatile oils.

Undesirable Side Effects

Too much green tea can be harmful: Excessive amounts can cause agitation, palpitations, or irregular heartbeat. Since large amounts of green tea can harm the liver, people with liver disease need to exercise caution.

How to Use Green Tea

When buying tea, choose vacuum packed products and purchase only small amounts to ensure freshness. Green tea loses some of its vitamins when stored for long periods of time. It should be kept in special tea tins in a cool, dry place.

Tea

Recipe

▶ *This is what you need:*
A teapot used exclusively for green tea that gets rinsed only with hot water, never with dish detergent; soft water; and tea.

▶ *This is how it's done:*
Fill the teapot with hot water to warm it up. Bring a quart of
water to a boil and let it cool off for five minutes. Never pour
boiling water over green tea. The ideal water temperature is
140 to 180 degrees Fahrenheit. Discard the water in the
teapot. Measure one level teaspoon of tea leaves per cup
into the pot and add hot water. Do not use tea "eggs" that
crowd the leaves together. Tea leaves should be able to
spread out well in the pot. Steep the tea for two to three
minutes. A shorter steeping time results in a tea that is more
stimulating, whereas a longer one (more than five minutes)
makes a more calming tea.

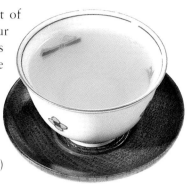

Tip

Reuse the Leaves for Several Batches
Never prepare more tea than you will drink within one hour.
If you empty the pot right away, you can leave the leaves
inside for later use. Depending on the variety, green tea leaves
can be reused up to four times. If the pot isn't emptied immediately, either remove the leaves or pour the brewed tea into a
second, pre-heated pot to keep it from turning bitter.

You will benefit most from the health promoting and mildly
stimulating properties of green tea if you drink about three large
cupfuls a day. Some Chinese scientists even recommend considerably larger amounts. If you are sensitive to caffeine, let your tea
steep longer or choose varieties that contain less caffeine. You can
also discard the first batch after steeping it for one minute.
Depending on your taste and on how the tea has affected you in the
past, steep the second and third batch for about three minutes.

Tea for Packs and Compresses

▶ Pour a quart of hot water over four teaspoons of green tea and
steep for five minutes. Strain the tea and chill it in the refrigerator.

Recipe

Green Tea Bath

▶ Fill your bathtub with slightly hot water (just under 100 degrees F).
Add a quart of very strong tea (steeped for about ten minutes).

Recipe

When to Use Green Tea

Green tea can be used for many purposes, especially for prevention of cardiovascular disease, cancer, and tooth decay.

Main Applications at a Glance

Ailments:	Suggested Applications:
Diarrhea	Drink at least a quart of green tea
Dry, stressed skin	Wash with green tea, drink tea regularly
Eczema; inflamed, irritated skin	Wash with green tea; green tea bath
Gingivitis	Use green tea as a mouthwash
Immune deficiency	Drink green tea regularly as a preventive measure
Loss of appetite	Drink green tea a half-hour before meals
Physical exhaustion	Drink up to a quart of green tea (with honey, if desired)
Sore throat	Gargle with green tea

Cardiovascular Disease and Cancer

Regular consumption of green tea can help prevent premature aging, cardiovascular disease, and cancer. If you have heart disease or cancer, continue to follow your doctor's instructions. Drinking green tea can be consumed along with standard medical treatment.

Recipe

▶ Drink at least two to three cups of green tea per day.

Mental and Physical Stamina

Green tea has a calming and mentally stimulating effect. It improves concentration and stamina. Drinking green tea is a natural way for athletes to enhance their physical fitness and obtain the minerals needed by the body.

Recipes

▶ *Mental and nervous exhaustion:*
Drink two to three cups of green tea per day. Enhance the beneficial effects of the tea by creating your own tea ceremony.
▶ *Physical exhaustion:*
Over the course of a day, drink about a quart of green tea; add some honey if desired.

Ailments of the Digestive Tract

The many minerals contained in green tea can benefit your entire body, beginning with your teeth. Due to its astringent effect, green tea alleviates inflammation of the mucous membranes of the mouth, stomach, and intestines. Green tea also stimulates appetite, relieves diarrhea, and replaces lost minerals.

Recipes

▶ *Dental cavities and gingivitis:*
Drink two to three cups of green tea per day, or use it as a mouthwash. Rinse several times a day for five minutes, especially at bedtime. This treatment is highly recommended for children.
▶ *Loss of appetite:*
Drink one to two cups of green tea half an hour before each meal.
▶ *Minor diarrhea:*
Drink at last a quart of green tea.

Sore Throat

Drinking green tea strengthens the immune system, and is therefore a great way to replenish fluids when you have a cold. The tannins it contains relieve sore throat.

Recipe

▶ At the first scratching sensation in your throat, gargle with very strong green tea for five minutes.

Skin

Due to its antioxidant properties, green tea can delay the aging process of the skin and help it retain moisture. Taken internally, its active ingredients make skin healthier from within and more resistant to external effects. Used externally, green tea is soothing, strengthens the skin's protective layer, protects against acids, and reduces inflammation. Tannins are responsible for the tea's astringent effect and make it an increasingly popular ingredient for skin creams.

Recipes

▶ *Eczema; inflamed, irritated skin:*
Wash the affected area with strong tea. Take a green tea bath once a week.
▶ *Sunburn:*
Apply soothing green tea compresses several times a day.
▶ *Dry, tired skin:*
Wash your face with cool green tea at mornings and evenings, if possible. Wash your entire body with cold green tea each morning.

Herbs and Spices

Healthier and Tastier Food

Apicius, the famous gourmet cook of ancient Rome, used some of the same spices we are all familiar with today—although in different combinations. Adding flavor to food, however, was not the only purpose spices were used for. Some of them played a role in religious rites, while others served as medicines.

Spices were also regarded as a symbol of wealth. They were expensive, since they were brought from far away and were subject to high taxes. Princes and wealthy merchants who used large amounts of spices to show off their wealth were known as "pepper sacks." For the wedding banquet of King Charles of Burgundy around the middle of the 15th century, the cooks were said to have used over 400 pounds of pepper! Catherine di'Medici finally halted this trend. She used her influence as a member of the French royal court to promote the idea that the individual flavor of foods should not be overpowered by spices. This marked the beginning of today's "haute cuisine."

Growing your Own Herbs

You can grow your own culinary herbs in your garden, or on a smaller scale, on your deck or porch. In any case, they will need a sunny spot in order to thrive. Plants grown on a deck or in a roof garden will require more watering because of the extra exposure to the sun, but they will do great.

Herbs need to be protected from the wind

Even if you don't have a garden or a deck, that doesn't mean you have to do without fresh herbs. Perennials, such as lemon balm, lavender, bay leaf, rosemary, sage, and thyme also grow very well on a sunny windowsill.

How to Plant Herbs

When buying seeds or seedlings, make sure that they are of good quality. Inferior plants or seeds are sometimes contaminated with germs or pests, which can spread throughout your herb garden. Also, some inferior varieties of herbs don't have much flavor.

Important! *Important:* Make sure that the seeds are spaced far enough apart, and thin out the plants before they grow too tall. When planting seedlings, give them enough room to grow.

Proper Care

You may not need to use any fertilizer in your garden if the ground is adequately mulched twice a year, usually around the end of April and again in the fall. Herbs grown in pots, however, need to be fertilized regularly—every three weeks or so—because their roots are confined to a small space, and the potting soil provides only a limited supply of nutrients. Organic fertilizers are the best choice.

Fresh herbs add such delicious flavor to your foods that growing them yourself is well worth the effort

In the spring, cut back the dried-up stalks of your perennials. Many herbs like bay leaf and rosemary are annuals and have to be transplanted and brought indoors before the first frost. Placed in a well-lit room and watered sparingly, they should make it through the winter in good shape.

How to Preserve Herbs

Fresh herbs are abundant throughout the summer. Some plants, like basil and chives, can be grown in pots on a windowsill during the winter months. Most other herbs need to be harvested by late fall and preserved by freezing, drying, or other methods. Freezing herbs is the best way to preserve their flavor.

Freezing

Most herbs, such as parsley, basil, dill, tarragon, chives, lemon balm, and thyme, can be frozen. After chopping the freshly picked herbs, put them into ice cube trays and fill the trays with water. Remove the frozen cubes and place them in larger containers or freezer bags for storage. You can also freeze herbs whole. Wrap them in aluminum foil and crush them in the foil before you use them.

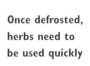

Once defrosted, herbs need to be used quickly

Drying

Culinary herbs can also be dried. This is best done in a dark room. Tie the herbs into bunches and hang them up in a dry, well ventilated place. Dried herbs retain their flavor for about a year.

Preserving with Salt, Italian Style

Place fresh leaves, such as basil, in layers into a jar or container. Lightly sprinkle each layer with salt and fill the container with enough olive oil to cover the herbs. Keep tightly closed in the refrigerator.

Preserving in Vinegar or Oil

Finely chop freshly picked herbs, put them into glass jars, and fill the jars with wine vinegar or oil.

How to Use Various Herbs and Spices

Anise
- sweet and spicy tasting seeds; goes especially well with ginger, cloves, nutmeg, and vanilla
- stimulates appetite, relieves indigestion and cramps, cuts mucus, stimulates secretion of gastric juices
- especially suitable for breads, Christmas baking, stewed fruit, vegetables, Asian meat dishes, in tea mixtures used for coughs

Caraway
- dark brown, crescent-shaped seeds with slightly sweet, aromatic flavor; tastes especially good with garlic, onion, and chili
- excellent antidote for gas; stimulates the secretion of gastric juices and bile, thereby helping to digest fats; relieves cramps
- important ingredient in stomach and gallbladder teas; ideal for flavoring foods that tend to cause indigestion

Chili
- fresh, dried, or pickled red pods, very spicy; because it lacks flavor of its own it can be combined with any other spice
- stimulates appetite, aids digestion, and improves blood circulation
- as a vegetable or spice for meat, soups, and sauces; for best results, cook along with the other ingredients; be careful not to add too much (1/2 pod for four servings)

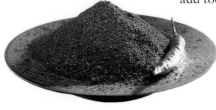

Chives
- tubular leaves with slightly spicy-aromatic, refreshing flavor; goes well with all other fresh herbs

- rich in vitamin C, stimulates appetite and aids digestion; lowers slightly elevated blood pressure
- used as a substitute for onion in soft cheese spreads and herbal butter, in soups and salads

Can be grown on a windowsill and used fresh even in winter

Cloves
- dried buds with intense, aromatic flavor and odor; goes especially well with cardamom, and cinnamon; can also be combined with bay leaf, pepper, and onion
- aids digestion, acts as an antiseptic and a pain reliever
- can be chewed to treat gingivitis, used as a breath freshener after eating garlic, as a flavoring in meat dishes, fatty fish, red cabbage, Christmas baking, fruit compote, and for pickling

Dill
- fresh leaves with intense, slightly sweet, aromatic flavor; flavor of seeds resembles caraway; can be combined with all fresh herbs but best when used by itself
- very rich in vitamin C, stimulates appetite, relieves minor cramps, stimulates milk production during lactation
- used in tea mixtures to stimulate milk production; leaves are added to salads, fish, white sauces, and sour pickles; seeds are used like caraway seeds

Fennel
- fresh leaves taste slightly like dill; goes well with dill, garlic, parsley, and onion; seeds taste similar to anise, yet not sweet
- relieves indigestion and cramps, cuts mucus
- used primarily to relieve indigestion and gas in infants; an ingredient in teas used to treat coughs; seeds used in breads, cakes and cookies, and in soups

Garden cress
- young shoots with pungent flavor resembling radish; because of its distinctive flavor it's best used only with pepper and onion
- stimulates appetite, aids digestion and kidney function, and acts as a diuretic
- for salads, as an herb added to soft cheese spreads, for herbal butter, as a flavoring for fish and soups, or as a topping on bread and butter

Cress is ideal for a spring cure

Ginger
- fresh, pickled (or, if necessary, dried) root with slightly sweet, pungent, spicy flavor; goes especially well with cardamom, coriander, cloves, and cinnamon

Gingerroot can be preserved by placing the peeled root in a jar with dry sherry or white rum

- stimulates appetite, cuts mucus, and promotes perspiration
- used as a flavoring in Indian dishes, for meat, salads, cakes, and fruit compote; should be cooked along with the food

Horseradish

- roots with pungent, mustard-like flavor; best combined only with garlic, pepper, and onion
- stimulates the secretion of bile, thereby helping to digest fat; has strong antibiotic properties
- used in poultices to treat neuralgia and rheumatoid arthritis; used in commercially available preparations to treat infections of the respiratory and urinary tracts; a flavoring for beef dishes and fish; do not cook with food

Juniper

- dried fleshy berries with bitter, resiny, very slightly sweet flavor; is best combined with other herbs such as fennel, garlic, bay leaf, marjoram, and parsley

Do not take during pregnancy or if you have kidney disease

- stimulates appetite, relieves indigestion, and acts as a diuretic; aids kidney function
- as a blood purifier when suffering from skin disorders, gout, or rheumatoid conditions; a flavoring for sauerkraut, meat, and fish; in herbal liqueurs and schnapps (gin); cook with food!

Lemon balm

- fresh or dried leaves with refreshing, lemony taste; can be combined with other fresh herbs

Lemon balm attracts bees

- stimulates appetite; relieves abdominal gas; has calming properties; reduces abdominal cramps; even acts as an antiviral agent
- used for nervous indigestion and nervous heart conditions (neurocirculatory asthenia); as an ingredient in calming teas and in ointments used to treat cold sores; a flavoring for salads, sweet dishes, and liqueur (lemon balm liqueur)

Marjoram

- fresh or dried leaves with strong, slightly minty flavor; goes well with sage and rosemary, but not oregano

Marjoram is best combined with only one other spice at a time

- stimulates appetite, helps digest fat, relieves gas and minor cramps
- used as an ingredient in teas that stimulate appetite and in ointments to treat colds in infants; counters gas; used primarily as a flavoring for fatty foods, such as roasts, stews, and sausages.

Mugwort
- dried buds with mild, slightly bitter flavor, goes especially well with onion, garlic, pepper
- stimulates appetite and the production of gastric juices and bile, which are both needed for digesting fats
- as part of a tea mixture used to treat stomach and gallbladder complaints, as a spice for fatty roasts or for vegetable dishes

Do not use mugwort during pregnancy

Mustard
- black mustard seed has a spicy-aromatic flavor; goes well with garlic, bay leaf, parsley, onion, and with many fresh herbs
- stimulates appetite and saliva production and blood circulation; combats bacteria and fungi; helps digest fatty foods
- as a powder for poultices to relieve pain of sore throats, pulled muscles, gout, osteoarthritis, and sciatica; seeds are used for pickling vegetables; the tips of fresh shoots are added to salads

Parsley
- leaves and root with slightly sweet to pungent, aromatic flavor; goes well with almost all other herbs
- fresh leaves are rich in vitamins A and C; stimulates appetite and the circulatory system; promotes digestive juices; improves kidney function
- parsley seeds are used in diuretic teas; parsley tincture is used to relieve earaches and rheumatoid conditions; a universal flavoring for salads, soft cheese spreads, vegetables, potatoes, meat, and soups; included in many herbal mixtures

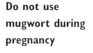

Peppermint
- fresh leaves with slightly sweet and peppery, refreshing flavor; used sparingly in combination with other herbs, it adds a refreshing twist to foods and beverages
- the menthol contained in the leaves acts as an antibacterial agent and a pain reliever; relieves minor cramps; stimulates appetite and the secretion of bile and gastric juices
- used as an ingredient in stomach and intestinal teas to relieve stomachaches, nausea, indigestion, feelings of fullness, gallbladder complaints, headaches, insomnia, and nervousness; a flavoring in meat dishes—do not cook, since it tastes best fresh

Use rosemary only
sparingly during
pregnancy

Rosemary
- needles and small sprigs with slightly resiny, bitter-aromatic flavor; goes especially well with garlic, thyme, and parsley
- its volatile oils and tannins stimulate appetite and nervous and circulatory systems
- used as a tea or in baths for treating exhaustion and weakness associated with aging; a flavoring for stews and for roasts

Sage
- fresh or dried leaves with a slightly pungent, bitter-aromatic, somewhat resiny flavor; due to its distinctive flavor, best used only in combination with garlic, pepper, and onion
- aids digestion, acts as an anti-inflammatory agent; reduces perspiration; strengthens nerves
- used in teas for gargling to relieve sore throat and to treat mouth infections; a flavoring for soups, stews, and meats

Savory
- fresh and dried stems and flowers with peppery, bitter flavor, goes well with bay leaf, parsley, rosemary, onion
- stimulates the secretion of gastric juices, relieves cramps, and cuts mucus
- as part of a tea mixture used to treat stomach complaints
- as a spice for wild game and legumes, or for quick and easy bean stews

Thyme
- fresh or dried leaves or young shoots have a slightly pungent, aromatic flavor that goes best with bay leaf, parsley, garlic, and onion
- its volatile oils relieve cramps; useful as an antiseptic agent and as an expectorant; stimulates appetite and the secretion of gastric juices
- used as a tea for cough and bronchitis; relieves gas and abdominal cramps; a flavoring for meat, stews, and vegetables, such as tomatoes, mushrooms, and eggplant

Do not take large
amounts of thyme
for extended
periods of time

Honey

A Sweet-tasting Nutrient and Remedy

Honey is much more than just a tasty food. It is a tonic that makes the body more resistant to all kinds of diseases, and it can be used as a remedy to aid in the treatment of many ailments. It may not be suitable for diabetics.

Ever since its discovery honey has been a much desired luxury food. There is evidence that people began collecting honey in pre-historic times. A 16,000 year old cave painting in the Spanish province of Valencia depicts a girl removing a honeycomb from a crevice, surrounded by a swarm of bees.

For preventing almost any ailment

The ancient Greeks used to drink mead, a fermented beverage made from honey mixed with water. Later, people discovered that wounds healed faster when covered with an ointment prepared from honey and clay. Honey has also been used in many cultures to treat infections and diseases of the eyes and the lungs. It is even said to enhance sexual potency. Do not give honey to an infant under one year of age because there is a slight chance the honey could be carrying botulism.

Honey Is Made from Nectar and Honeydew

Bees use either nectar, the sweet liquid produced by flowering plants, or honeydew from the forest to make honey. Honeydew is contained in the leaves and needles of trees. Tree-dwelling insects, such as aphids, whose diet consists of leaves and needles, excrete the

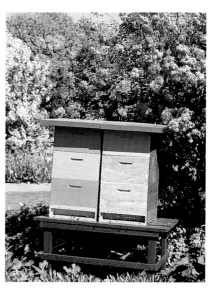

sugary liquid. Using their proboscides, field bees collect the nectar and honeydew, mix it in their crops with enzymes, and bring it back to their hives. There, they regurgitate it and turn it over to hive bees, who add saliva and more enzymes. The resulting raw honey is filled into honeycombs where it is thickened by evaporation. The beekeeper uses a centrifuge to extract the honey from the combs.

Hives where bees store their honey

Why Is Honey So Valuable?

The contents, the taste, consistency, color, and smell of honey vary from one type to another. It mainly contains fructose and grape sugar or glucose; glucose is quickly absorbed into the bloodstream and provides an immediate boost of energy. Fructose, however, is stored in the liver for later use. Unlike refined sugar, honey doesn't just provide empty calories without any useful nutrients. It contains enzymes needed for the synthesis of certain inhibitors, which, along with other chemically active compounds found in honey, prevent the growth of various bacteria and fungi. Honey is low in acids, a property that further enhances its antibacterial effect.

Honey does not just provide empty calories, but many valuable nutrients

Honey is not a major source of vitamins and minerals, providing only small amounts of various B vitamins, sodium, calcium, and magnesium. However, it is rich in trace minerals, especially iron and zinc. It also contains several constituents resembling hormones. One of them, acetylcholine, promotes the uptake of glucose into the muscles and also regulates blood pressure and heart rhythm.

Undesirable Side Effects

Be careful if you are allergic to pollen

You needn't anticipate any side effects from honey. It may, however, aggravate diarrhea, and should therefore be used only sparingly in that instance. The pollen in honey may rarely cause an allergic reaction.

How to Use Honey

Due to the presence of heat-sensitive enzymes, honey should not be heated above 104 degrees Fahrenheit. If crystallized, it can be liquefied by immersing the jar in warm water. Honey is sensitive to light, and it easily absorbs moisture and odors. It is therefore advisable to store it in a tightly closed container in a dark place.

Honey can be eaten plain by the spoonful, dissolved in tea, or otherwise added to foods.

Important!

Important: Do not take large amounts of honey (two to six teaspoons) all at once. Instead, divide it into several doses taken throughout the day. Let it slowly dissolve in your mouth.

Let honey dissolve slowly in your mouth

In Germany, specially prepared honey is sometimes administered by injection to provide a source of immediately available energy. This is done only by qualified health care professionals, and only after it has been established that the patient is not allergic to pollen.

Processed honey is added to various commercially available preparations, such as cough syrups.

When to Use Honey

Honey acts as a general tonic, has a calming effect on the nervous and circulatory systems, relieves cold symptoms, and soothes irritated or infected skin.

Main Applications at a Glance

Ailments:	Suggested Applications:
Acne	Facial mask, or apply to pimples
Allergies, asthma	Honey cure
Cold, flu, bronchitis, cough, sore throat	Eat plain or add it to tea for colds
Constipation	Eat plain or dissolve it in laxative tea
Decreased heart function	Eat honey regularly
Digestive problems	Eat plain or add it to digestive tea
Failure to thrive, lack of concentration	Honey cure
Immune deficiency	Honey cure
Infections	Honey cure
Injuries and wounds	Apply honey
Sleep disorders	Dissolve honey in sedative tea
Loss of appetite	Eat honey
Nervousness	Honey cure; for acute conditions, eat plain
Physical or mental exhaustion	Honey cure

Physical and Mental Exhaustion

Power food for the physically weak or for competing athletes

Honey is a great tonic and energy booster and can help build up strength in people who are generally exhausted, chronically fatigued, or lacking in stamina. A honey cure quickly restores a patient's energy after surgery or a long illness. The simple sugars (monosaccharides) contained in honey are a source of immediate energy to the body because they are absorbed directly into the bloodstream in their original form. Other active ingredients found in honey provide steady, sustained energy after the initial boost.

Recipe ▶ If you feel weak and exhausted, such as after surgery or a long illness, take four or more teaspoons of honey daily until you feel better. Eucalyptus, heather, peppermint, and mixed flower honeys are best. For milder cases, a teaspoonful mornings and evenings is sufficient.

Decreased Heart Function

Honey has a strengthening and healing effect on the heart as well. It increases blood flow to the coronary vessels that supply the heart muscle with oxygen and nutrients. It provides acetylcholine, which further enhances the functioning of the heart. This makes honey especially beneficial for people whose heart function is decreased due to aging, a long illness, or smoking. Honey is also an ideal tonic for the elderly.

Recipe ▶ For a honey cure, take four or more teaspoons of honey daily for three weeks. If possible, use honey made from the nectar of hawthorn flowers. Eucalyptus, heather, peppermint, or a mixed flower honey are next best. After three weeks, the dosage can be reduced to a teaspoonful taken morning and evening.

Insomnia and Lack of Concentration

Honey whisks make removing honey from jars easy

People who often feel irritable, restless, or stressed, and who suffer from insomnia or lack of concentration can all benefit from taking honey. It supplies the body with calcium, phosphorus, magnesium, and the "nerve vitamins" of the B group, which all have a calming effect on the nervous system.

▶ *Nervousness:*
Drink two to three cups of a calming tea per day. Add one teaspoon of honey per cup. Lemon balm or orange honey are best.

▶ *Insomnia:*
Prepare a calming tea that promotes sleep and add a teaspoon of honey, preferably linden, lemon balm, or orange honey. Drink one or two cups half an hour before bedtime.

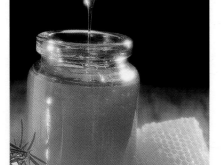

Infections

Honey acts like a broad-band antibiotic. It contains inhibitors that kill bacteria and inhibit infections. Honey is no substitute for a real antibiotic, of course, but it can easily be used as a supplement.

▶ *Bacterial infections:*
If you suffer from a cold, flu, urinary bladder infection, or any other infectious disease caused by bacteria, take four teaspoons of honey a day. For fever or cough, use either linden flower or tree honey if available. Acacia, heather, lavender, cabbage flower, and peppermint honey are also good choices. Note, however, that these types of honey are not readily available, and may have to be obtained through mail order sources.

After the infection is gone, keep taking one or two teaspoons of honey per day for another three weeks in order to strengthen the immune system. For chronic bronchitis, take six teaspoons of honey daily for four weeks.

▶ *Sore throat, cough:*
Unless the respiratory pathways are severely congested, slowly sip a glass of warm milk with a teaspoon of honey mixed in. Honey added to lemon juice is also excellent for soothing sore throats.

Recipes

Detoxifying the Body

Honey detoxifies by stimulating bile production and liver function. It thus helps to eliminate toxins from the body, strengthing the immune system and improving general health.

▶ Take a honey cure in the spring and again in the fall. Take two or three teaspoons of honey daily for about six weeks. You can dissolve the honey in two or three cups of stinging nettle tea.

Recipe

Digestive Problems

Honey is very easily digested due to the fact that most of its sugars do not need to be broken down further in the intestine. This eliminates fermentation. Honey acts as a mild laxative, stimulates appetite, and regulates the production of stomach acid. Taken regularly, it relieves nervous indigestion and alleviates diarrhea caused by bacteria.

▶ Before meals, and in between, if needed, take a teaspoon of honey either plain or dissolved in a tea prepared to relieve indigestion. Acacia, lemon balm, and peppermint honey are recommended for digestive problems.

Recipe

Allergies

Some people experience an allergic reaction to honey or to the pollen it contains. Symptoms include diarrhea, rashes, hay fever, or even asthma. On the other hand, honey can relieve existing allergies, even those caused by pollen. It seems that by strengthening the immune system honey can also help prevent allergies.

Recipes

▶ *Pollen Allergy:*

Take a teaspoon of mixed flower honey, preferably collected in your vicinity, every day. Proceed with caution and watch for reactions. If symptoms don't get worse within a few days, continue taking a teaspoonful of honey daily.

▶ *Asthma:*

Take six teaspoons of honey daily for four weeks.

Minor Wounds, Injuries, and Infections

Honey is also helpful for treating wounds and injuries. It contains antiseptic agents that can prevent wound infection. Honey tends to attract moisture. Applied to wounds, it draws out blood and lymphatic fluid and promotes healing. Honey also has a cooling effect and reduces pain.

Recipes

▶ *Minor cuts and injuries:*

Apply a thick layer of honey to the injured area. Cabbage flower, lavender, and peppermint honeys are best. Wrap the area with a gauze bandage or, even better, allow it to dry uncovered.

▶ *Blemished, infected skin:*

Apply a thick layer of honey to clean facial skin. Remove with water after half an hour. Clean thoroughly. Dab individual pimples with honey several times a day. In addition, eat one teaspoon of honey per day, preferably acacia, cabbage blossom, or peppermint honey.

Honey for Children

Babies under the age of one year should not be given honey, since their intestinal flora are not yet stable. In rare cases that could lead to life-threatening infant botulism, a type of food poisoning. Honey could also increase the risk of allergies. For all other age groups, honey is perfectly appropriate. It increases appetite and protects against intestinal disorders and infectious diseases, stimulates blood production, and provides various minerals. It's also food for increasing stamina and relieving fear of failure caused by poor concentration in school. Of course it also contains lots of sugar, so children should not forget to brush their teeth after eating honey.

**Important!
Do not give
honey to
babies under
the age of one**

▶ *Failure to thrive and poor concentration:*

Children should be given one to three teaspoons of honey depending on their age, but should not be given to children under the age of one year.

Kefir and Kombucha

Healing Drinks for Everyday Use

Kefir and Kombucha are two fermented beverages that taste refreshing, are stimulating, and are said to promote beauty and longevity. While until recently they were enjoyed primarily in Russia, their use is now spreading throughout the entire world. Both the Kefir grain and the Kombucha mushroom ferment liquids—milk or tea—with microorganisms that benefit from each other.

Kefir

The people of Central Europe have known how to ferment milk for hundreds of years. Some time ago, the inhabitants of the Caucasus mountains, where Kefir originates from, drew international attention because so many of them live to be 100 years old or even older. Around the end of the 19th century Kefir clinics were established throughout Russia. They admitted patients suffering from various ailments, such as gastrointestinal, lung, and gynecological disorders, rickets and anemia, as well as people who needed to recuperate after a long illness.

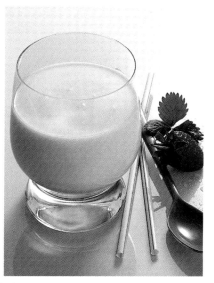

Kefir and fruit taste great together

Kombucha

This special beverage, made with black, green, or herbal tea, was discovered by a Korean physician by the name of Kombu, who used it to cure the emperor of Japan of a stomach disease around 400 A.D. Thus kombu-cha, the tea of Kombu, became famous throughout the world. Before World War II Kombucha was known and widely used in Germany as a beverage and a remedy. After falling into disuse for a while, it is now regaining popularity: Madonna, Daryl Hannah, and Linda Evans all either drink a glass of Kombucha every day or apply pieces of the miracle mushroom as a facial mask each morning.

What Kefir and Kombucha Look Like

Kefir

The Kefir culture is an organism resembling a miniature cauliflower. It consists of soft, translucent white grains made of a cartilaginous substance; it is used to turn cow's, sheep's, or goat's milk into a refreshing effervescent beverage. Kefir cultures reach a size anywhere from about a half-inch in diameter to as large as a child's fist. They are an efficient micro-laboratory consisting mainly of lactic acid bacteria and yeasts. The cultures turn lactose into lactic acid and help break down casein, or milk protein, into easily digestible amino acids, producing B-vitamins, carbonic acid, and alcohol in the process.

The greater the culture content, the stronger the taste of the Kefir and the higher the nutritional value

Kombucha

The "tea mushroom" is also a symbiosis of acid bacteria and various yeasts. It is grayish-white in color and looks like a thick pancake with a consistency varying from mucous-gelatinous to tough and leathery. Put into a liquid, it spreads over the entire surface of its host. Bacteria cause the growth of gelatinous cellulose. They use the metabolic products of the yeasts for energy, while the yeasts feed on the bacterial products, namely gelatin and acid. The microorganisms turn the sugar added to the tea into acetic acid, lactic acid, alcohol, and carbon dioxide.

How to Make Your Own Kefir and Kombucha

Kefir

The Kefir culture turns milk into a refreshing carbonated drink. Depending on how long it is left in the milk to ferment, the resulting beverage is either mildly acidic or tastes quite sour. With proper care, a Kefir culture will keep growing small granules that can easily be separated from the main grain to be used as new starters.

Recipe

▶ *This is what you need:*
Three-quarters of an ounce of Kefir culture, a quart of pasteurized milk, a glass jar with a wide mouth, and a lid

▶ *This is how it's done:*
Rinse the jar with hot water, using no detergent. Pour the milk into the jar, leaving room for the culture. Add the culture to the milk and close the lid. Store the jar away from light at a temperature of about 77 degrees Fahrenheit (no higher than 86 or lower than 41 degrees) for one to two days. Shake occasionally during the fermenting process. When done, strain the Kefir through a sieve to filter out all the culture. Finished Kefir stays fresh in the refrigerator for up to fourteen days. If you like strongly carbonated Kefir, let the mixture ferment for less than twenty-four hours at a temperature of about 83 degrees. When not in use, Kefir cultures can be stored in distilled water in the refrigerator for about twenty days.

Do not wash the culture. Residual lactic acid helps preserve it

Kombucha

Kombucha turns tea into a slightly acidic, aromatic, delicious, and refreshing drink that resembles apple cider in flavor and helps digestion. Depending on the fermenting conditions, such as room temperature and length of time the starter is left in the tea, and the individual culture and how quickly it works, the resulting Kombucha can taste from fruity and refreshing to slightly sour.

▶ *This is what you need:*

A large glass, porcelain, or clay jar (a glass preserving jar that holds two to three quarts of liquid will do fine), a quart of black, green, or herbal tea, two-and-a-half ounces of honey or sugar, about four fluid ounces of previously fermented tea, Kombucha culture, a thin cloth or paper tissue, a rubber band, and several bottles for storing the finished drink.

▶ *This is how it's done:*

Prepare a quart of tea as described earlier in the book. Let the tea steep for fifteen minutes, then strain it and allow it to cool to room temperature. Dissolve two-and-a-half ounces of honey or sugar in the tea. Rinse the jar with hot water (do not use detergent) and pour the mixture into it. Add about four ounces of previously fermented Kombucha tea. Carefully introduce the gelatinous Kombucha culture on top of the liquid. Cover the jar with a thin cloth or one layer of paper tissue and secure it with a rubber band. Make sure that a sufficient amount of oxygen can pass through. Store in a well-ventilated place protected from bright light, at a temperature of about 73 degrees Fahrenheit, and allow to ferment. After seven to ten days, remove the culture and store it temporarily in a small, covered container. Strain all but about four ounces of the fermented liquid into bottles and store them in the refrigerator. Wash the Kombucha culture under running cold to lukewarm water, and store it in the liquid you have set aside in the fermenting jar for when you make the next batch.

With sufficient warmth, the culture will grow and replicate itself after about ten days. You can also propagate the culture by dividing it: simply pour a mixture of equal parts of fresh tea and fermented drink into a second jar, and add a small piece of Kombucha culture. It should form layer of new starter a quarter- to a half-inch thick within three to four weeks.

As new layers form, they can be used for starter

Recipe

When the culture sinks to the bottom, a new layer will grow on the surface of the tea

How Kefir and Kombucha Work

Kefir

We do not yet fully understand all the mechanisms of how Kefir works in the body, but we do know the following: to begin with, Kefir contains the active ingredients of the milk that was used. Bacteria and yeasts provide additional amounts of B vitamins and improve the intestinal flora. Carbon dioxide and alcohol are produced during fermentation, but only in small amounts comparable to those found in nonalcoholic beer. Lactic acid bacteria inhibit harmful fermenting processes in the intestines. This, among other actions, may have earned Kefir its reputation as a source of health and longevity. To enjoy these benefits, you need to consume at least eight ounces of Kefir a day.

Carbon dioxide and alcohol content are the same as in Kefir

Kombucha

Sugar (glucose, fructose), lactic, glucuronic and other acids, vitamins, enzymes, chemical compounds that act like antibiotics, carbon dioxide, and small amounts of alcohol can all be found in Kombucha. When consumed regularly, this drink cleanses the body of toxins, stimulates metabolic function, strengthens the immune system, and keeps the intestinal flora healthy. Kombucha tea acts as a mild disinfectant and laxative and is said to be helpful in treating various ailments. It relieves fatigue and nervousness and is also used for more serious conditions, such as gout, rheumatoid disorders, arteriosclerosis, gastrointestinal problems, high blood pressure, and immune deficiency.

Undesirable Side Effects

Kefir

Kefir can decrease the effects of some prescription drugs and should therefore not be taken along with, but rather either two hours before or after these medications. People on blood thinners should take no more than one glass of Kefir a day, since Kefir can interfere with the effect of those drugs.

In cases of immune deficiency, keep everything very clean

Kombucha

This tea beverage has no side effects. However, possible contamination of the culture with harmful germs could pose a risk for anyone, especially for people with immune deficiency. Pay special attention to cleanliness and good hygiene. During fermentation, the cover on your jar should allow oxygen to pass through, but at the same time protect the tea from dust and insects. Do not use cultures that have been around too long (those that form a very thick layer or are dark in color).

How to Use Kefir and Kombucha

● Ready-made Kefir

Ready-made, commercially produced Kefir contains little culture and tastes more like sour milk so it will suit Western palates. It's better to brew your own Kefir since you can prepare it the way you like it.

● **Kefir culture**

If you know people who make their own Kefir, ask for a piece of their culture. Or you can order a small grain through the mail.

● **Freeze-dried fermenting agent**

This is an option if you find it too inconvenient to care for and maintain a Kefir culture. The resulting drink tastes similar to freshly cultured Kefir. The fermenting agent comes in packages that make about ten to fifteen batches of Kefir each.

 Tip

Kefir for Your Cereal
Use Kefir instead of milk on your breakfast cereal. Eaten together with whole grains and fruit, it makes a complete, nutritious meal.

Kombucha

Kombucha is also produced commercially, but it is relatively expensive to buy. You are better off making your own. Get a culture from someone you know or order a piece from a supplier.

When cared for properly, the culture stays viable indefinitely

When to Use Kefir and Kombucha

You shouldn't drink Kefir and Kombucha only when you're sick. These fermented drinks can help your body even when you are healthy.

Main Applications at a Glance

Ailment:	Suggested Applications:
Arteriosclerosis	Kombucha or Kefir cure
Gastrointestinal complaints	Kombucha or Kefir cure
Gout	Drink Kombucha or Kefir regularly
Immune deficiency	Drink Kombucha or Kefir regularly
Infections	Drink Kombucha or Kefir regularly
Rheumatoid conditions	Drink Kombucha or Kefir regularly
Seasonal fatigue	Kombucha or Kefir cure

Tip When making your first batch of Kombucha, use sugar instead of honey, since honey can damage the culture.

Gastrointestinal Complaints

Kefir is an ideal drink for people with lactose intolerance

Kefir and Kombucha restore your intestinal flora to health. They contain lactic acid bacteria that crowd out harmful microorganisms in your intestines and provide an ideal environment for beneficial bacteria to grow.

Carbon dioxide and lactic acid, as well as the slightly bitter taste of both beverages, stimulate appetite and aid digestion. Kefir and Kombucha can both prevent and cure infections of the mucous membranes that line the gastrointestinal tract.

Detoxifying the Body, Chronic Conditions

Kefir and Kombucha help the body excrete metabolic waste products and toxins. This makes them ideal remedies for seasonal fatigue, gout, and rheumatoid conditions. When taken regularly, both drinks are said to be useful in treating arteriosclerosis and hypertension. Kombucha also relieves pain and reduces inflammation.

Recipe ▶ Drink one or two glasses of Kefir or Kombucha daily.

Infections

Both Kefir and Kombucha strengthen the immune system, and Kombucha directly inhibits the growth of bacteria. If a serious condition makes taking antibiotics necessary, Kombucha can help prevent side effects such as unhealthy intestinal flora.

Recipe ▶ While taking antibiotics, drink a glass of Kefir two hours after the morning dose and two hours before the evening dose of your medication. Following treatment, drink three glasses of Kefir daily for another three to four weeks.

Cancer

Kefir and Kombucha may help prevent breast and colon cancer.

Recipe ▶ Drink two to three glasses of Kefir or Kombucha per day.

Onions

For Flavor, Prevention, and Healing

For over 5000 years, the onion has been used in various cultures as a vegetable, a spice, and a remedy. The Egyptian workers who built the pyramid of Khufu were fed large amounts of leeks and onions to keep them healthy and increase their stamina. The ancient Romans advocated the use of white onions as an aphrodisiac and as a means to increase sexual potency. Old herbalists praised the medicinal properties of the onion and recommended it as a treatment for coughs, rheumatoid conditions, heart disease, dog bites, and all kinds of congestion. Onions were grown for medicinal use in the gardens of medieval monasteries. In recent decades, scientific research has confirmed the health benefits of eating onions. In spite of that, the kitchen onion hasn't yet earned a spot in medical schools.

Flowering onions

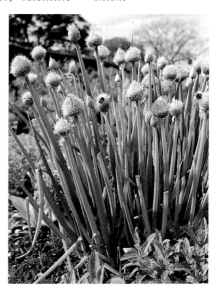

The Different Varieties of Onions

The culinary onion (*Allium cepa*) can be either an annual or a perennial. The onion bulb with its many fleshy leaves is really a reservoir of nutrients for the plant's large, purple flowers. The green, tubular tops can reach a height of almost three feet. There are many varieties of onions with bulbs of various sizes, colors and flavors, from white to purple, and from mild to sharp.

- The common yellow onion tastes pungent and spicy and can be stored for months.
- The sweet onion, used as a vegetable, has a very mild flavor. It is grown mostly in Spain and can grow to be very large.
- The spring onion also has a mild flavor. It is sold and used together with its tops and can be stored for only a few days.
- The white onion is very juicy and has a sharp taste. It can be stored for about two weeks.
- The red onion is also very juicy and has a mild, spicy flavor. It goes bad much more quickly than the yellow onion.
- Shallots are a noble variety of onion with an especially delicate, aromatic flavor.

Cultivating and Harvesting Onions

A cool, dark, dry place is ideal for prolonged storage of up to several months

Onions love sunny locations and loose, rich soil that hasn't been freshly fertilized. They self-propagate either through seeds or bulbils. The easiest way to grow them is through small bulbs called sets. Planted in the spring, the set will produce bulbs ready for harvest by August. You can tell that your onions are ready to be picked when the tops are dry. Pull out the entire plant, tie several tops together, and hang the onions up in bunches to dry.

What Makes Onions So Effective

Onions aid digestion and affect the body's metabolism

Like garlic, onions contain sulfur compounds. They are also an excellent source of flavonoids, minerals and trace minerals, vitamin C, and the B vitamins.

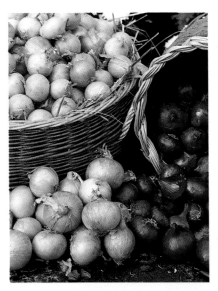

By promoting the secretion of gastric juices, onions stimulate appetite. The fiber they provide protects the mucous lining of the stomach. Onions have diuretic, antibacterial, and anti-inflammatory properties and act as an expectorant and pain reliever. Eaten regularly, they can lower slightly elevated blood pressure, inhibit blood clotting, and latch onto and destroy free radicals. This reduces the risk of heart attacks, strokes, and coronary disease. Onions also lower the blood levels of harmful lipids such as cholesterol; this is another benefit to the cardiovascular system. Onions may also reduce blood sugar.

How to Use Onions

In general, red onions taste milder than white onions, but they spoil faster

Although onions retain most of their active ingredients even when they are cooked or fried, it's best to eat them raw to ensure that none of the valuable vitamins are destroyed. Whether you use onions to prevent or to treat certain ailments, you should consume about two ounces of fresh onions per day for maximum health benefits. You can simply add half a medium-sized onion to your daily diet, either by chopping it into small pieces and eating it plain, or by adding it to salads, sauces, or vegetable dishes.

Syrup

This preparation is especially suitable for children. The addition of honey enhances the syrup's beneficial effects. Remember, do not give honey to children under one year of age.

Recipe

▶ *This is what you need:*
a medium-sized onion, three tablespoons of honey, and 1/2 cup of water
▶ *This is how it's done:*
Finely chop the onion and mix in the honey. Add the water and heat everything in a double boiler. Let steep for at least three hours, then strain. Take five to ten teaspoons throughout the day.

Onion Milk

Recipe

▶ *This is what you need:*
one small onion, one cup of milk, and one teaspoon of honey
▶ *This is how it's done:*
Finely dice the onion, mix it with the milk in a saucepan, and simmer the mixture over low heat for about five minutes. Remove from the heat, let steep until the milk is cool enough to drink, then strain and add a teaspoon of honey. If the breathing passages are congested with excessive mucus, substitute water for the milk.

Inhaling

Inhaling steam rising from cooked onions can irritate the mucous membranes of the nose. Therefore, inhale only briefly, and repeat the procedure later if necessary.

Recipe

▶ *This is what you need:*
one medium-size onion, a quart of water, and a large hand towel
▶ *This is how it's done:*
Add the finely diced onion to the water and cook it in a saucepan for two minutes. Let it cool slightly. Put the saucepan on the table. Position your head over the rising steam and drape the hand towel like a tent over your head and the saucepan. Inhale for about five minutes.

Onion Preparations

Some health food stores and herb suppliers sell onion preparations such as juice, or capsules containing onion powder.

Homeopathic Remedies

Allium cepa is the onion's homeopathic agent. It is often used to treat colds involving runny nose and eyes, and earaches.

When to Use Onions

Onions are mainly used to treat colds and to prevent ailments associated with aging.

Main Applications at a Glance

Ailments:	Suggested Applications:
Abdominal gas	Eat onions or take onion syrup
Bronchitis, Asthma	Inhale, eat onions, or take syrup
Constipation	Eat onions or take onion syrup
Cough	Drink hot onion milk
Earache	Apply a warm or cold ear pack
Geriatric ailments	Eat onions or take onion syrup
Insect stings	Apply a slice of onion
Lack of appetite	Eat onions or take onion syrup
Sore throat	Drink hot onion milk
Urinary bladder infection	Apply a warm onion pack

Diseases of Modern Civilization

Regular consumption of onions, like that of garlic, may help prevent cardiovascular problems associated with aging. Used to supplement conventional medical treatment, onions are also helpful in treating existing disorders. They also are effective in regulating the body's metabolic functions and may help reduce the risk of cancer. In regions of the world where people eat lots of onions, there are fewer cancer cases affecting the stomach, colon, esophagus, and lungs.

Recipe

▶ As a preventive measure, eat at least half a raw onion per day, or take five tablespoons of onion syrup.

Digestive Problems

Onions can relieve various digestive ailments. They stimulate appetite, improve digestion, and promote healthy intestinal flora, which is a prerequisite for a strong immune system.

▶ Anyone suffering from loss of appetite, constipation, or abdominal gas should eat half an onion or take five tablespoons of onion syrup over the course of a day.

Recipe

Respiratory Ailments and Earaches

Turn to the onion for relief from the symptoms of the occasional common cold. Onions are an effective home remedy for sore throats and coughs. Onions may help asthmatics by inhibiting spasms of the bronchi, thereby preventing asthma attacks.

Children are especially prone to earaches. A warm onion pack applied to the ear quickly relieves pain and reduces inflammation.

Recipes

▶ *Asthma, Bronchitis:*
Eat at least half an onion or take five tablespoons of onion syrup per day. To relieve persistent congestion, inhale the vapor from hot onions.

▶ *Sore Throat, Cough:*
Drink a glass of onion milk every day.

▶ *Earache:*
For earache, apply a pack with steamed onions up to three times a day (page 159).

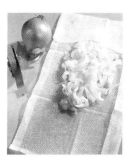

Urinary Bladder Infection

If you experiencing pain on emptying your bladder or feel a constant need to urinate, you probably have an urinary bladder infection. By applying a warm onion pack to your abdomen, you can use the pain-relieving and anti-inflammatory properties of the onion to alleviate your symptoms. But if the condition doesn't improve by the next day, you must consult your doctor.

✚ See a doctor

▶ At the first sign of a urinary bladder infection, apply a warm onion pack to your abdomen twice a day (see page 161).

Recipe

Insect Stings

Bee or wasp stings are painful and often cause considerable swelling. Onions are very effective in reducing swelling and itching.
▶ Place a thick slice of onion on the affected area immediately after you have been stung.

Recipe

Vegetable Oils

Prevention and Healing with Oils

Vegetable oils, especially olive oil, have a long history. The oldest preserved olive presses date back more than 7000 years, and the practice of extracting oil from olives may have had its beginnings several thousand years before that. In ancient times, olive oil was very popular throughout the Mediterranean regions. Owners of olive groves enjoyed prestige and wealth. Oils for cooking, perfumes and medicinal purposes were exported to places as far away as Egypt. Massaging the body with oil was customary. When asked about the secret to his longevity, the philosopher Democritus (550 A.D.) replied: "Honey used internally, oil used externally." For many

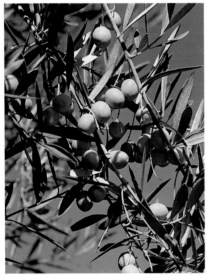

Olives on a tree

centuries, oil was the most important source of fat. It also found use in various rituals. In Israel, for instance, kings and priests were anointed with scented oil. Vegetable oils have been used as remedies in Ayurvedic medicine for a long time. In Russian folk medicine, sunflower oil is an ingredient in oil cures that people take to detoxify their bodies. Even modern Western medicine has finally acknowledged that adding certain vegetable oils to your diet can reduce the risk of heart attacks.

Vegetable oils are also used as bases for paints and stains, as lubricants for machines, for heating, and as fuel.

How Vegetable Oils Are Produced

Most vegetable oils are cold-pressed mechanically. This gentle process ensures oil of very high nutritional value, since most of the valuable active ingredients of the plant are preserved. Eleven pounds of olives yield a quart of pure olive oil. This oil is called "extra virgin" or "virgin." When buying oil, make sure that it has been cold-pressed.

Refined oil may stay fresh longer than unprocessed oil, but excessive heat and the use of chemical solvents have destroyed valuable nutrients, such as vitamins, flavonoids, and lecithin, as well as the oil's natural flavor and aroma.

Vegetable Oils

Oil	Characteristics	Active Ingredients	Benefits
Almond oil	an especially precious oil, light- to golden-yellow color, tastes slightly sweet, is excellent for sweet dishes and desserts	rich in vitamins A, B, E, and minerals	stimulates appetite, fights infections, acts as an expectorant, relieves dry skin, good for baby care, can be used as a laxative for children, is a good base for volatile oils
Canola oil	very mild, almost neutral flavor, good substitute for olive oil, since its active ingredients are very similar, tolerates heat	rich in mono-unsaturated fatty acids, large amounts of vitamin E	useful for treating liver and gallbladder ailments, regulates fat levels in the blood, prevents excessive stomach acid, protects cells, good for skin care
Corn oil	golden-yellow color, strong, somewhat peculiar flavor, do not heat	very rich in unsaturated fatty acids, vitamin A, B, E, minerals, and lecithin	inhibits cell damage, well suited to skin and hair care
Grape-seed oil	pale yellow to greenish color, sweetish flavor	very large amounts of polyunsaturated fatty acids, very rich in certain flavonoids that are more potent than vitamin E	protects against arteriosclerosis, prevents premature aging and cell damage, strengthens the immune system and connective tissues, thins the blood, a good massage oil
Linseed oil	dark-yellow color, some-what peculiar, slightly bitter flavor Tip: Tastes good in soft cheese spread served with potatoes	especially rich in unsaturated fatty acids	relieves gastrointestinal complaints by protecting the mucous membranes and acting as a mild laxative; has calming properties, helps with respiratory ailments and gallbladder colic; aids in wound healing and clears up eczema
Olive oil	yellowish to dark green in color, strong flavor, easily digestible, tolerates heat, but use refined olive oil for frying	rich in monounsaturated fatty acids, large amounts of essential fatty acids and vitamin E	useful for treating liver and gallbladder ailments, regulates fat levels in the blood, prevents excessive stomach acid, protects cells, good for skin care
Pumpkin seed oil	greenish-dark brown color	large amounts of vitamin E and phytosterols	reduces benign enlargement of the prostate, improves bladder function, inhibits infections, strengthens muscles and connective tissues
Sesame oil	mild, nutty flavor, bright- to dark-yellow color	rich in mono- and poly-unsaturated fatty acids, trace minerals, antioxidants and lecithin	especially useful for people with high blood pressure or diabetes, or those who have suffered a heart attack or a stroke, good massage oil, also said to be an aphrodisiac

Vegetable Oils

Oil	Characteristics	Active Ingredients	Benefits
Soy oil	orange-yellow color; use up within two or three months after opening a bottle	especially rich in vitamin A, E, and lecithin, contains large amounts of poly-unsaturated fatty acids	protects against cell damage, regulates fat levels in the blood, acts a nerve tonic
Sun-flower oil	light-yellow color, nutty flavor	very rich in vitamins A, E, and lecithin, large amounts of polyunsaturated fatty acids, additional substances	protects against cell damage, acts as anerve tonic, relieves gallbladder andliver ailments, acts as an expectorant, is a good massage oil, traditionally used in oil cures
Thistle oil	golden-yellow color, slightly nutty flavor, should not be heated	especially rich in poly-unsaturated fatty acids and vitamin E	regulates cholesterol levels, prevents atherosclerosis and cell damage, well suited to skin care
Walnut oil	light yellow color, nutty flavor, easily oxidizes when exposed to air, especially suitable for sweet dishes	very rich in poly-unsaturated fatty acids, rich in minerals and various vitamins	protects against arteriosclerosis, acts as a nerve tonic
Wheat germ oil	pleasant, grainy flavor	exceptionally rich in vitamin E, very large amounts of poly-unsaturated fatty acids	protects against cell damage and premature aging, aids in cell regeneration, softens skin, helps in scar healing, midwives recommend it for massaging the peritoneal area for several weeks before a delivery

What Makes Vegetable Oils So Valuable

The body needs saturated and unsaturated fatty acids

Fat is an important part of our diet; we can't live without it. It provides fuel for energy and plays a vital role in cell production. Fat also protects our nerve cells. Fatty acids facilitate the absorption of oxygen into the cells. Our bodies need them to produce proteins, enzymes, and hormones. There is, however, a significant difference between animal and vegetable fats: While they both contain saturated fatty acids, vegetable oils are a much richer source of mono- and polyunsaturated fatty acids than animal fats.

Unlike animal fats, vegetable oils are free of cholesterol yet rich in healthy nutrients, such as fat soluble vitamins (especially A and E), minerals, trace minerals, and lecithin. These oils increase the levels of healthy fats in the blood (HDLs, or high density lipoproteins) while reducing harmful fats (LDLs, or low density lipoproteins). In so doing, they lower the risk of arteriosclerosis and cardiovascular disease. Vegetable oils strengthen the immune system, aid metabolic function, and can prevent minor depression due to hormonal changes during menopause and before the onset of a woman's menstrual period.

Herbs added to vegetable oils provide a distinctive flavor

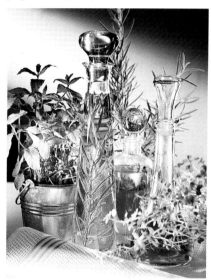

How to Use Vegetable Oils

Important: Depending on the variety, most cold-pressed, pure vegetable oils tend to oxidize and turn rancid easily. For this reason, it is important to use them up quickly once a bottle has been opened. Rancid fat contains harmful chemical compounds that can be harmful to health.

Cold-pressed vegetable oils should never be heated to high temperatures, since excessive heat can turn some of their originally very valuable constituents into carcinogens. Since refined oils no longer contain many of their desirable active ingredients, it makes more sense to use those oils for frying. It is a good idea to serve lightly sauteed vegetables or fresh salads made with cold-pressed vegetable oils along with fried, grilled or deep fried foods. These oils contain antioxidants that reduce the health risks inherent in eating heated oils and animal fats.

Never heat cold-pressed vegetable oils to high temperatures!

Oils Used in Cooking

Use unrefined, nutritionally valuable vegetable oils as often as possible to enrich raw vegetable dishes, salads, soups, and desserts. For cooking, frying, or baking, refined olive oil is a good choice since it remains relatively stable even when heated.

Plain or Added to Vegetable Juice

Taking plain vegetable oil may not sound very appetizing at first, but it is a good way to provide your body with a sufficient amount of polyunsaturated fatty acids. A daily dosage of two tablespoons is both safe and effective, and can be taken over long periods of time. If you can't bring yourself to swallow oil by the spoonful, you can add it to a glass of vegetable juice. The oil will improve the absorption of fat-soluble vitamins contained in the juice.

Oil Cure

An oil cure is recommended mainly for respiratory problems and head ailments, but it can also be used to treat any other condition stemming from an accumulation of toxins in the body, such as susceptibility to infections, various skin ailments, joint problems, and mild depression or insomnia.

An oil cure should last at least 4 weeks

The cure should last at least four weeks. Sometimes, results can be felt after only a week. Chronic conditions require a longer oil cure, whereby the procedure described below is repeated several times a day.

Recipe

▶ *This is what you need:*
Cold-pressed, organic sunflower oil, an egg carton or paper towels for disposal of the used oil

▶ *This is how it's done:*
Put a tablespoon of cold-pressed, organic sunflower oil (or another vegetable oil of comparable nutritional value) into your mouth and swish it through your teeth. Keep doing this for at least ten minutes. The recommended time is twenty minutes. After you are done, do not swallow the oil, which by now should be very diluted by saliva, but spit it out into the old egg carton or into a paper towel. Do not pour the oil into the sink, since fat causes problems for water treatment plants! The oil now contains large amounts of toxins and a lot of bacteria that would be easily visible under a microscope. Rinse your mouth with warm water and brush your teeth.

Do not pour the used oil into the sink

Massage Oil

Recipe

▶ *This is what you need:*
Olive, thistle, or almond oil (or any other oil made from nuts), essential oil, such as orange, lemon, or lavender

▶ *This is how it's done:*
Add a few drops of the essential oil to a mixture of one part olive, one part thistle, and one part almond oil. Warm the oil slightly,

apply it liberally to the skin, and massage it in. Remove any excess oil with a paper towel.

Leftover massage oil can be kept for several months in a tightly closed dark bottle.

Bath Oil

▶ *This is what you need:*
A quart of whole milk, three tablespoons of olive oil, your favorite aromatic oil
▶ *This is how it's done:*
Add whole milk, olive oil and a few drops of the aromatic oil to the running bath water. Instead of milk you can use buttermilk. It will leave your skin very soft.

Recipe

When to Use Vegetable Oils

Vegetable oils are used mainly for their ability to regulate cholesterol levels in the blood, and for other diseases commonly associated with our modern diet and life style. They are also beneficial for the digestive system and the prostate. Vegetable oils help the skin retain moisture and make it less susceptible to infections.

Main Applications at a Glance

Ailments:	Suggested Applications:
Constipation in children	Take cold-pressed vegetable oils
Dry, sensitive skin	Use massage and bath oil made with vegetable oils
Elevated cholesterol levels	Use cold-pressed vegetable oils for cooking, or take them plain
Enlarged prostate	Use pumpkin seed oil regularly
Gallbladder ailments	Take olive or other cold-pressed vegetable oils
Liver disorders	Use cold-pressed vegetable oils in cooking or take them plain
Over-processed hair	Massage scalp with almond, wheat germ, or corn oil
Stomach complaints	Take olive or other cold-pressed vegetable oils
Urinary bladder infection	Use pumpkin seed oil regularly

Diseases of Modern Civilization

People who regularly use vegetable oils lower their risk of many diseases. Unsaturated fatty acids and other valuable nutrients contained in these oils are known to play a role in preventing arteriosclerosis, high blood pressure, digestive problems, liver and gallbladder ailments, and diabetes. It is critical to have a proper diagnosis by a medical professional if you suspect you have any of these conditions, or other health problems. Due to their significant antioxidant properties, cold-pressed vegetable oils may help prevent premature aging and possibly even reduce the risk of developing cancer.

Recipe

▶ Include sufficient amounts of cold-pressed, unrefined vegetable oils in your daily diet. Take an oil cure on a regular basis, for instance in the spring and in the fall.

Digestive Problems

Vegetable oils stimulate appetite and aid digestion. They coat the mucous lining of the intestinal tract with a protective layer, reduce inflammation, and act as a mild laxative. Since they increase the secretion of bile, they are used to treat liver ailments and gallstones.

Recipes

▶ *Liver and gallbladder ailments:*
For acute conditions, take two tablespoons of olive oil. For chronic disorders, take two tablespoons of either olive, linseed, or sunflower oil per day, either plain or added to foods.
▶ *Stomachache, heartburn, gastritis:*
Take two tablespoons of vegetable oil, preferably on an empty stomach.
▶ *Constipation in children:*
Give your child up to four teaspoons of almond oil.

Benign Enlargement of the Prostate and Bladder Irritation

Phytosterols, obtained from pumpkin seeds, play a role in healthy prostate and urinary bladder function. Pumpkin seed extracts especially formulated for treating benign enlargement of the prostate are commercially available. To enhance the beneficial effect of these supplements, you can include additional pumpkin seed oil in your diet. This oil is also helpful in treating bladder irritation, a condition that mainly affects women and is characterized by a persistent, painful urge to urinate and impaired urinary flow.

Recipe

▶ Take one to two tablespoons of pumpkin seed oil per day, or simply use an equivalent amount on a regular basis in raw vegetable dishes and salads.

Skin and Hair Care

Vegetable oils useful in regular skin care for restoring moisture to dry skin. They are also recommended for treating certain chronic dry skin conditions. The valuable active ingredients found in these oils are absorbed into the skin and make it more supple, improve circulation, and help the skin get rid of toxins. They can also help revitalize overtreated hair. Regular treatments with oil restore luster to dull hair and prevent split ends.

▶ *Dry, sensitive skin:*
Apply a massage oil to the affected area on a regular basis. Avoid commercially available bubble baths and soaps. Instead, use an easy-to-prepare bath oil (see page 60).

▶ *Dry, rough skin on hands or feet:*
Pour a small amount of almond, grape seed, wheat germ, or olive oil, or a mixture of several of these oils, into the palm of one hand. You can add a drop of your favorite essential oil if you wish. Massage the oil for about ten minutes into each finger, the palms, the backs, and the wrists of your hands (or the toes, soles, and insteps of your feet). Afterwards, remove any excess oil with a paper towel.

▶ *Overtreated hair:*
Before going to bed, massage some almond, wheat germ, or corn oil into your hair, especially the ends of your hair. Cover your pillow with a large towel! Shampoo your hair as usual in the morning.

Recipes

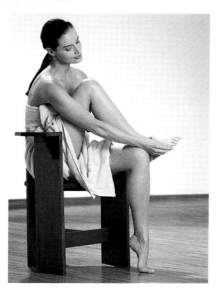

Moisturize your skin regularly with massage oil

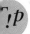
A Treat for Your Hands and Feet
Massage vegetable oil into your hands and/or feet before you go to bed at night. Wear cotton gloves and/or socks afterwards. Your skin will be wonderfully soft and supple in the morning.

White Cabbage and Sauerkraut

A Delicious Treat for Your Intestines

Sauerkraut has had a long-standing reputation as one of the healthiest foods we know. It is enjoyed both by people who prefer simple, home-style cooking and by those with a more sophisticated palate. In the Alsace, where sauerkraut is a national food, it has a permanent place on the menus of expensive gourmet restaurants. Although it is commonly thought of as a typical German food, the French and the Americans actually consume more sauerkraut than the Germans.

Sauerkraut probably originated in Asia. We know that the ancient Greeks and Romans prepared it and used it as a remedy. The cabbage varieties grown in Central Europe today were brought to Germany via France by Roman legions. On his voyage around the world, Captain James Cook carried sauerkraut aboard his ships to protect his crews from scurvy, a disease caused by a deficiency in vitamin C. Sebastian Kneipp, a German priest and healer who lived in the 19th century, used to prescribe a cup of raw sauerkraut or sauerkraut juice taken on an empty stomach for various ailments, such as sluggish bowel, stomach ulcers, worms, gout, and diabetes. He treated wounds and open sores with sauerkraut juice or cabbage-leaf packs. Cabbage eaten in salads and raw sauerkraut are also said to relieve bronchitis, eczema, sciatic pain, phlebitis, and rheumatoid conditions.

Quality and Ingredients

Cabbage is one of the oldest cultivated plants

Sauerkraut is made from white cabbage (*Brassica oleracea*). Specific varieties of the plant that produce firm, white heads weighing up to about fifteen pounds each are used to prepare this popular food. Sauerkraut made from *Filderkraut*, a variety of white cabbage with elongated, pointed leaves, is considered to be a special Swabian delicacy. Various ingredients are usually added to sauerkraut to enrich its flavor. The recipe for wine sauerkraut, stemming from the Alsace region, calls for at least two quarts of grape or apple wine per 220 pounds of kraut. Gourmet sauerkraut is prepared with carrots, caraway, and mustard seeds, juniper berries, and pieces of apple.

Good quality sauerkraut is always pale in color, crisp, and free of any tough, soft, or woody pieces of cabbage. It is not supposed to contain any parts of the head's tough core or any large, uncut leaves, and it should smell slightly sour.

How Sauerkraut Is Made

Among the major regions where white cabbage is grown are Swabia, which produces the delicious *Filderkraut*, Hesse, Schleswig-Holstein, the Lower Rhine regions, Lower Bavaria, and of course Alsace. After the cabbage heads are harvested, the coarse outer leaves and the core are removed. The inner leaves are cut into strips and placed in evenly salted layers into a barrel. The shredded cabbage is compressed with a vibrating device. A plastic bladder or sac filled with water is laid on top to provide an airtight seal. Cabbage juice extracted by the salt drives out any remaining air. Lactic acid bacteria start the fermenting process and reproduce at a rapid rate. Their presence crowds out any undesirable bacteria that could cause spoiling.

After fermenting for one to three weeks (the time varies depending on the season and temperature), the sauerkraut is heated in a vat to 194 degrees Fahrenheit in order to get rid of carbon dioxide. It is then packaged and heated once more to 201 degrees Fahrenheit to pasteurize it.

Pasteurized sauerkraut stays fresh for as long as four years

What Makes Sauerkraut So Effective

White cabbage is rich in many valuable nutrients, such as vitamin C, vitamin B2, potassium, calcium, and iron. It is also a good source of dietary fiber. The fermenting process produces B12, a vitamin otherwise rare in vegetables and vegetable products. Lactic acid bacteria deprive undesirable bacteria like molds and yeasts of their food by turning fructose and starches into lactic acid and carbon dioxide. After the sauerkraut has been consumed, these beneficial bacteria continue their action in the human gastrointestinal tract. They destroy harmful germs, improve the health of the intestinal flora, and aid digestion. Lactic acid helps break down proteins, is mildly laxative, strengthens the immune system, and has anti-inflammatory properties. Eating sauerkraut significantly reduces your risk of developing colon cancer.

Sauerkraut is low in carbohydrates and calories, but at the same time very filling. This makes it an ideal food for people who want to lose weight. It also helps prevent diseases associated with overweight, such as high blood pressure and arteriosclerosis. Sauerkraut

Healthy intestinal flora and a low pH in the intestine significantly reduce the risk of intestinal cancer

is also one of the best natural remedies for gastrointestinal problems, and it seems to lower blood sugar. Many diabetics swear by it and use it regularly in their diet.

Unwanted Side Effects

Sauerkraut with potatoes relieves heartburn

People with a sensitive stomach shouldn't cook sauerkraut with fat or meat. Flavor it with spices such as caraway seeds, fennel, juniper berries, and honey. Add sausage links, lard, meat, or bacon only at the very end.

How to Use White Cabbage and Sauerkraut

Chewing sauerkraut thoroughly allows saliva to start the digestive process

Sauerkraut is most nutritious when eaten fresh and uncooked. When packaged in plastic bags, it quickly loses some of its vitamin C. Since fermentation continues even in the refrigerator, sauerkraut cannot be stored for long. Opened packages must be kept in the refrigerator, with enough brine to cover the kraut. Don't discard the brine. It contains valuable nutrients. You can use the leftover liquid in soups.

Fresh and Raw

Raw sauerkraut tastes delicious eaten plain or added to a salad. In this form, it is richest in vitamin C and most effective as a remedy.

Pasteurized Sauerkraut

Delicious in soups, casseroles, or used as a filling

Sauerkraut sold in cans has been pasteurized. This process destroys the lactic acid bacteria and some of the vitamin C, but not the B-vitamins and minerals. Pasteurized sauerkraut may not be as nutritious and healthy as raw sauerkraut, but it is still considered a valuable food.

Sauerkraut Juice

Sauerkraut juice is refreshing and has an spicy flavor. A glass taken in the morning aids digestion and supplies important nutrients to the body.

Cabbage Juice

Cabbage leaves can be put through a juicer. Although the resulting juice tastes rather bland, it is very beneficial for the mucous lining of the gastrointestinal tract.

Cabbage Leaf Packs

▶ Remove the large veins from a few young cabbage leaves. Soften the leaves by rolling them with a rolling pin or a bottle. Steam the leaves lightly over boiling water by placing them over the rim of the pot. You can also cut a tender young leaf into small strips and stack them in a roofing-shingle pattern on the affected area. Hold the leaves in place with a loosely tied gauze bandage. The pack needs to be changed morning and evening. Rinse the wound each time with lukewarm chamomile tea.

Recipe

Make sure that the pack doesn't exert any pressure. Secretions must be able to escape

When to Use White Cabbage and Sauerkraut

The gastrointestinal tract and the skin benefit most from remedies that use white cabbage.

Main Applications at a Glance

Ailments:	Suggested Applications:
Arteriosclerosis	Eat sauerkraut regularly
Burns	Cabbage leaf pack
Constipation	Drink sauerkraut juice, eat sauerkraut
Gastritis, gastric ulcers	Take a cure with cabbage juice
Immune deficiency	Take a sauerkraut cure
Intestinal infections	Drink sauerkraut or cabbage juice
Overweight	Take a sauerkraut cure
Shingles	Cabbage leaf pack
Varicose ulcers	Cabbage leaf pack

Immune Deficiency

If you want to strengthen your immune system, lose a few pounds, or do something beneficial for your gastrointestinal tract, you should take a sauerkraut cure.

▶ Eat a portion (four to eight ounces) of raw sauerkraut, prepared to taste, twice a day between meals for three to four weeks.

Recipe

Gastrointestinal Ailments

Gastric ulcers heal quicker in patients who drink cabbage juice on a daily basis. Pain and heartburn usually disappear within a few days. Cabbage juice is also helpful for treating intestinal infections.

Sauerkraut juice is a tried-and-true home remedy for constipation. Regular consumption of sauerkraut may help prevent intestinal cancer.

Recipes

▶ *Stomach ulcers:*
Drink a quart of cabbage juice per day for four to five weeks. The juice is meant to supplement a light diet and should be taken after meals.
▶ *Intestinal infections:*
Drink sauerkraut or cabbage juice regularly. For acute conditions, take up to a quart per day.
▶ *Constipation:*
Drink one or two glasses of sauerkraut juice every morning before breakfast. Eat sauerkraut with meals or as a snack.

Diabetes, Arteriosclerosis, Overweight

Sauerkraut regulates sugar and fat levels in the blood. It is useful as part of a weight loss diet, and is also ideal for people with dietary restrictions due to illness.

Recipe

▶ Eat raw sauerkraut at least once or twice a week. Every now and then, take a sauerkraut cure by eating two portions (four to eight ounces) of sauerkraut a day.

Skin

Due to its valuable active ingredients, sauerkraut nourishes the skin from within. Used topically in the form of packs, cabbage leaves are effective in treating varicose ulcers, a condition caused by poor circulation in the legs. By drawing out liquid and puss, cabbage packs promote wound healing. Infected skin rashes, such as shingles, and minor burns also heal faster when treated with cabbage leaf packs.

Recipes

▶ *Varicose ulcers:*
Prepare cabbage leaves as described on page 71. Clean wound thoroughly with lukewarm chamomile tea, then apply the cabbage leave pack. Keep it loosely in place with a gauze bandage. Change the pack twice daily.
▶ *Shingles, minor burns:*
Apply a cabbage leaf pack as described on page 71. Keep it loosely in place with a gauze bandage. Change the pack twice a day.
▶ *Infected wounds:*
For infected minor wounds, apply a pack of small cabbage leaf strips arranged in a roofing-shingle pattern.

Wine

Red Wine Helps Prevent Heart Attacks

Wine has always had a special meaning for mankind. It has been associated with pleasure, with health, and with the supernatural. "Wine will comfort and sustain us through the trials and hardships of this earth," Noah's father told him. Guided by these words, Noah started to cultivate grapes as soon as he left the arc. Jesus is said to have turned water into wine.

Since ancient times, wine has also been used to treat various ailments. Often, medicinal herbs were added to wine and administered in that fashion. This practice served a dual purpose. The alcohol in wine preserved the herbs, and it also made the medicine more palatable. Hippocrates recommended wine for many uses: as a tonic, a sedative and sleep aid, a disinfectant, a pain reliever, for headaches, indigestion, and for cardiovascular ailments. Over the last decades, research has confirmed the health benefits of wine for the heart. Studies have found a significantly lower incidence of cardiovascular disease among people living in Mediterranean countries than in those living in central and northern Europe. This difference has been attributed to the regular consumption of red wine, as is the custom in Mediterranean regions. However, wine contains alcohol, and there seems to be a fine line between healthy and unhealthy amounts of alcohol in the diet.

There are about three-and-a-half ounces of alcohol in quart of wine

Why Is Wine So Effective?

All in all, more than a thousand different chemical substances have been identified in various wines. Each wine is unique, depending on the grapes that were used, the region where they were grown, and the specific climatic conditions during a given season. The specific amounts of these substances and their combination give each wine its distinctive flavor, color, and aroma.

Each quart of wine contains about three-and-a-half ounces of alcohol, along with sugar, minerals, trace elements, vitamins, various acids, tannins, and aromatic chemical compounds. Red wines in particular are also rich in antioxidants, especially polyphenols. These valuable chemical compounds can also be found in large amounts in fruit and vegetable juices. In that form they are not very stable, but the alcohol in wine preserves them.

Wine Protects Against Certain Diseases

Alcohol helps reduce cholesterol and improves blood circulation

People who regularly consume moderate amounts of wine are not only less likely to suffer from coronary heart disease, but they also generally live longer than nondrinkers. Alcohol helps reduce cholesterol levels, acts as a blood thinner, and improves circulation. This increases the flow of oxygen to the brain, which may help slow down the deterioration in brain function associated with age. However, since regular consumption of other alcoholic beverages doesn't have the same effects on circulatory function, the health benefits of wine do not appear to be attributable to alcohol alone. They are probably due in large part to one or more of the other chemical compounds found in wine.

Drinking moderate amounts of red wine on a regular basis reduces the risk of heart attack

Wine also increases appetite and aids digestion. It inhibits the formation of kidney stones and seems to lower the risk of cancer. Drinking moderate amounts of wine reduces the effects of stress on blood vessels and nerve cells. It also lowers insulin and increases estrogen levels in the blood. Aged white wine in particular acts as a disinfectant and is helpful in preventing diarrhea.

Why Wine Drinkers Feel Better

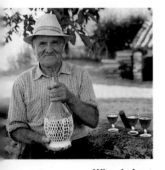

Wine can improve a person's mood just like coffee, tea, or sweets. As little as one glass is enough to boost self-confidence and produce a sense of well-being. This is due to the effect alcohol has on serotonin, a neurotransmitter that is known to enhance mood. Like light and exercise, alcohol inhibits the breakdown of serotonin in the brain. Too much wine, however, can have the opposite effect. It can cause restlessness, anxiety, and insomnia.

Wine is best consumed with food

Consumed regularly and in moderation, wine offers more advantages than disadvantages. Some wine experts even hold that abstinence from alcohol constitutes a health risk!

Why Men Tolerate More Wine than Women

Alcohol is broken down in the body by an enzyme called alcohol dehydrogenase (ADH). This compound is found mainly in the liver, but also in the stomach. Women produce smaller amounts of ADH and have less body mass than men. This makes them more sensitive to alcohol. The degree of chemical activity of ADH varies from person to person. The same amount of alcohol can therefore produce different blood alcohol levels in different people.

Alcoholic beverages are less harmful for both genders when taken with meals. Food causes alcohol to remain in the stomach longer, and gives the ADH more time to break it down.

Undesirable Side Effects

If you have ever had too much wine, you know of its undesirable side effects firsthand. The symptoms of a hangover are due to by-products that accumulate when alcohol is broken down in the liver. Regular alcohol abuse over an extended period of time can cause abnormal fatty deposits in the liver, hepatitis, cirrhosis of the liver, and chronic inflammation of the pancreas. It also destroys brain cells, slows down reactions, and increases the risk of certain kinds of cancer.

Drinking too much alcohol is even more dangerous when combined with an inadequate diet

Certain wines, mostly the cheaper varieties, contain various chemical substances that can cause problems in sensitive individuals. Sulfur, added in small amounts to most wines as a preservative, sometimes produces allergic reactions. The same is true for histamine, which can also cause headaches, palpitations, and hot flashes. You should stop drinking a wine if you experience any of the above symptoms. Sometimes fusel oils, found in some of the most expensive wines, are responsible for undesirable side effects. Some people experience irregular heartbeat after drinking a certain wine. Switching to another variety may eliminate this problem.

Since alcohol increases the production of uric acid, it should be consumed only sparingly, if at all, by people who have gout. Pregnant women should avoid alcohol, especially during the first trimester. People with liver disease and women with increased risk of breast cancer should also abstain from alcohol.

What Kinds of Wine, and How Much?

Red wine probably has slightly higher health benefits than white wine, but, it has not been proven conclusively which wine is healthier.

Most wines contain between eleven and thirteen percent alcohol per volume. Wine that is twelve percent alcohol contains 120 milliliters of alcohol per liter, which is about 100 grams (a milliliter of alcohol weighs .8 grams). There are about seventy grams of alcohol in a .7 liter bottle of wine. The optimum daily allowance of alcohol is 24 grams for women and 32 grams for men. This is equivalent to .3 liters and .4 liters of wine, respectively. Or putting it more simply: a couple can share a bottle of wine for dinner, and the man can have a slightly larger share than the woman.

Vary the kinds of wine you drink

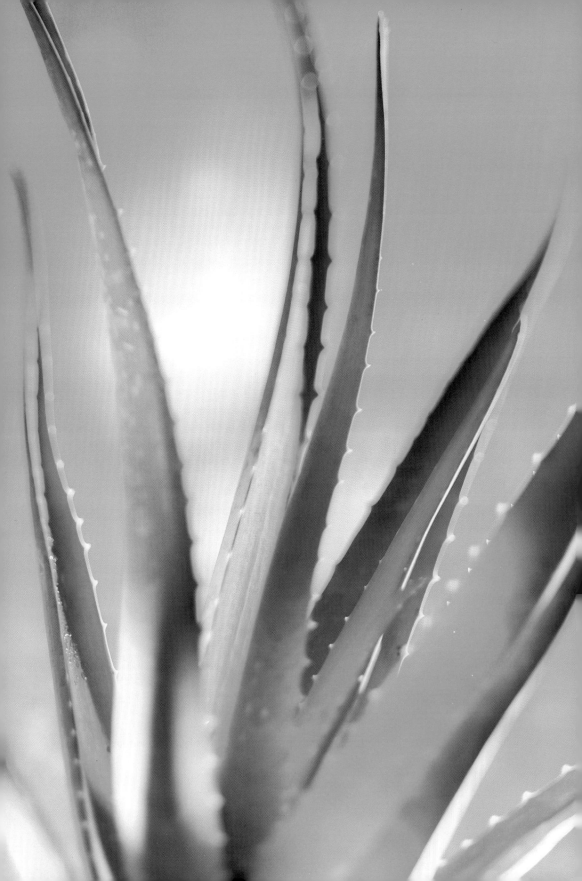

The Best Herbs

Herbal preparations are enjoying great popularity, and are being prescribed by many natural healers and alternative health practitioners. Herbs promote healing—there is no doubt about that. We now have scientific proof that they are effective. Many herbal preparations are equivalent or even superior to certain synthetic chemical drugs. A case in point is St. John's wort, an herbal remedy whose effectiveness in treating mild to moderate depression is as good as that of synthetic antidepressants. What's more, St. John's wort causes virtually no side effects.

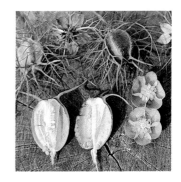

Treating yourself and your family and friends with home-grown herbs is very enjoyable. Herbs cultivated in your own garden or on your deck or porch contain the same amounts of active ingredients as those purchased in a health food or natural food store, provided you use high quality seeds, plant them in a sunny spot in good soil, and give them adequate fertilizer. A tea brewed from fresh leaves always tastes better than one made from dried leaves. In this chapter, you will learn which herbs can be useful for various ailments, and how you can grow and use them.

Herbs for Everyday Use

The most common and the oldest way to use herbs is to prepare a tea by pouring hot water over the dried parts of the plant. Not every tea works in the same way, however, so it sometimes matters whether a certain herbal tea is taken before or after a meal, and whether it is sweetened or not. Tea can also be used externally for treating wounds in the form of partial baths, wraps, or washings.

There are many herbs that can't be made into tea; others require special methods to unlock their active ingredients. Alternative methods of extraction, such as steam distillation or steeping in alcohol, may be required to make use of these herbs.

Cultivating and Harvesting Herbs

Many herbs can easily be grown in your own garden or on your deck or porch. One advantage of using home-grown herbs is that you know they have not been sprayed with pesticides. Trying to protect your plants from air pollution, however, may be a harder, if not impossible, task. As each herb is introduced in the following chapters, you will find instructions on how to grow it successfully.

Before you collect any herb in the wild, make sure that it isn't endangered and protected by law

If you decide to collect herbs in the wild, you should have a good knowledge of the plants you are looking for. Avoid areas where plants are likely to be contaminated with chemical residue, especially those in close proximity to heavily traveled highways, industrialized areas, and fields where crops are sprayed with weed killers and pesticides.

The Right Time to Harvest

As a rule, herbs should be picked on dry, sunny days. Whole herbs are usually harvested shortly before they bloom, and flowers are collected immediately after they open, in midmorning as soon as the dew has evaporated. Ripe seeds are best picked early in the morning, since that's when the seed heads are less likely to lose their seeds. Fruits are harvested when they are fully ripe. Mature roots and rhizomes should be dug out either in the spring or in the fall. Bark is cut from young shoots in the spring.

Except for the roots, herbs should not be washed

How to Preserve Herbs Properly

After they are harvested, herbs must be dried quickly and as carefully as possible. They keep losing some of their active ingredients even after drying, so they should be used within a year.

Drying: Tie herbs into small bunches and hang them up to dry in an airy room away from direct sun. When the leaves rustle and the stems are brittle, the herbs are completely dry. Wash harvested roots thoroughly, cut them into pieces about an inch long, and dry them in your oven at low heat (about 135 degrees Fahrenheit).

Storage: Store dry herbs in dark glass jars or in wood or tin containers that can be tightly closed to keep out any moisture.

Remember to label your jars

The Main Active Ingredients Found in Herbs

An herb usually contains one or several active ingredients responsible for its main therapeutic action, along with many other less important chemical constituents that together account for its overall medicinal effect. In addition to carbohydrates, fats, proteins, and fiber, there are secondary compounds that act as coloring, protection against pests and diseases, or hormones to regulate growth. Each of these constituents can have either beneficial or detrimental effects on the human organism. Two examples of chemical compounds that are detrimental to human health are hydrocyanic acid, a chemical present in uncooked legumes, and solanin, found in the green parts of the potato.

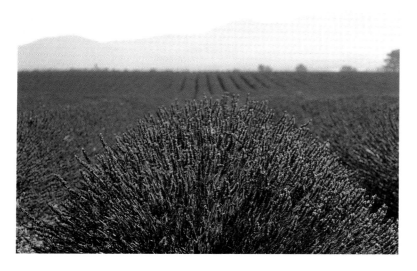

Lavender is an herb that contains volatile oils

Alkaloids

Most herbal toxins, such as atropine found in deadly nightshade, morphine in poppies, or colchicine in autumn crocus, are alkaloids. Medicinal use of these substances requires their isolation from the plant, thereby permitting administration in very precise doses.

Bitters

Bitters aid digestion

These chemical compounds promote the production of gastric juices and bile, thereby stimulating the appetite and aiding digestion. Bitters also strengthen the heart and the circulatory and immune systems. They increase overall well-being.

Glycosides

Flavonoids and glycosides have anti-inflammatory and diuretic properties

In addition to flavonoids, there are two other chemical compounds that make up the group of glycosides. They are saponins and phenylglycosides. Most plants contain flavonoids. This type of glycoside can produce a number of different effects, depending on the specific flavonoid and on the amount present in the plant. Flavonoids almost always contribute to an herb's general medicinal properties. They can act as antioxidants, anti-inflammatory agents, or diuretics. Plants containing flavonoids also relieve cramps and regulate blood circulation, especially in the capillaries. Hawthorn, arnica flowers, birch leaves, the seeds of lady's thistle, and other herbs contain flavonoids.

Saponins suspended in water produce a soapy foam when shaken. They cut mucus and are used to treat coughs. Saponins reduce inflammation, lower cholesterol levels in the blood, and have diuretic properties. They facilitate the absorption of other active ingredients in the intestines. Ivy leaves, ginseng, legumes, oats, some vegetables, and the roots of primrose and licorice contain saponins.

Phenylglycosides are found in herbal laxatives made from senna leaves, rhubarb root, and the bark of alder buckthorn.

Inorganic Substances

Many herbs also contain various trace minerals, such as potassium, sodium, and silicic acid. Plants belonging to the horsetail, borage, or grass families (such as bottle brush or shave grass) absorb large amounts of silicic acid from the soil. Silicic acid is essential for the formation of human connective tissue, skin, hair, and nails.

Mucilage

These polysaccharides form a soft protective layer on mucous membranes and reduce irritation, relieve coughing, and act as a mild laxative. Flax, hollyhock, Iceland moss, and marshmallow contain significant amounts of mucilage.

Mucilage relieves irritation

Tannins

Tannins bind to proteins in human skin and mucous membranes. In so doing, they rob of their nutrients any bacteria that have invaded injured skin or mucous membranes. Tannins reduce irritation and inflammation. Herbs rich in tannins are used in gargling solutions to soothe sore throats, in mouthwashes to reduce gingivitis, in compresses applied to wounds, and as remedies to relieve diarrhea. Bloodroot or tormentil, oak bark, and blueberry contain large amounts of tannins.

Tannins reduce irritation and inflammation

Vitamins

Vitamins are essential for the health of the human organism. While some of them can be manufactured by the body, many must be obtained from food. Vitamins are the main active ingredients in common sea buckthorn and rose hips.

Volatile Oils

A large number of plants contain strongly scented, very volatile oils whose function is to protect the plant from parasites, fungi, and loss of moisture due to evaporation. These oils are extracted by steam distillation.

Used externally, herbs rich in volatile oils, such as St. John's wort or black cumin, reduce inflammation and improve blood circulation, but they can also irritate the skin. When taken internally, these oils act as decongestants and expectorants, improve gastrointestinal, liver and gallbladder function, relieve cramps, and have diuretic and antiseptic properties.

Undesireable Side Effects

Certain herbs, such as arnica flowers, mistletoe leaves, or psyllium seeds, cause allergic reactions in some people. Some sensitive people can get headaches from teas made with herbs rich in tannins or bitters. Laxative herbs should not be used for extended periods of time because they can cause a deficiency in essential electrolytes such as potassium.

Unwanted side effects can occur due to allergies, particular sensitivities, or excessive dosage

How to Use Herbs

Herbs are used either internally or externally, depending on the preparation. Most herbs are taken as teas. Two external applications, wraps and compresses, will be discussed in a separate chapter that begins on page 152.

Tea

● **Coarsely chopped herbs** are commercially available from health food and natural food stores. They can be bought in bulk and mixed as desired.

Mixtures must be shaken or stirred before being used, since small, lightweight particles tend to settle.

● **Tea bags** offer the advantage of always having convenient portions of pre-measured herbs at hand. Since the herbs in tea bags are cut into tiny pieces, their active ingredients can be released easily. This can, however, also be a drawback, especially with respect to volatile oils. They dissipate quickly when the cells that hold them are destroyed. The amount of volatile oils in teas, especially those sold in grocery stores, is therefore often below the required minimum. Low quality tea products can also contain parts of the herb that provide no active ingredients, such as stems and leaves of the chamomile plant in addition to its flowers.

Don't buy low quality tea, and check manufacture or expiration dates

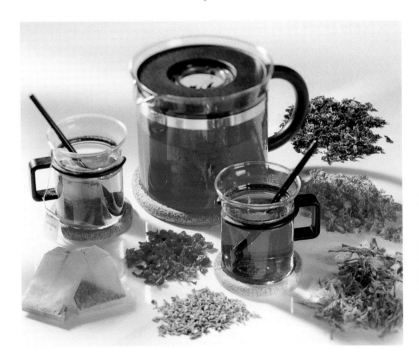

Tea made with dried herbs and with tea bags

● **Instant teas** are easy to prepare since they don't require steeping or straining. The active ingredients of the herb have been extracted with water and alcohol, an ideal medium to dissolve a broad spectrum of chemical compounds. Instant teas are available in powdered or granular form. Granules often contain added sugar, but you can buy sugar-free products especially formulated for diabetics and children.

How to Prepare Teas

With few exceptions, teas are best consumed in the morning on an empty stomach, in the afternoon, or at bedtime. A tea cure should last about three to four weeks. As a rule, herbal teas should not be combined with over-the-counter medications or prescription drugs since they can reduce the effectiveness of the tea.

● *Infusion* is the most commonly used method of preparing tea. It is especially suitable when using an herb's flowers, leaves, or entire tops.

▶ Pour hot water over the dried herbs. Let steep for five to ten minutes, then strain.

Recipes

● *Maceration* (cold water extraction) is used for plants rich in mucilage (such as marshmallow root, flax or psyllium seeds, and hollyhock) or herbs containing an excessive amount of tannins (such as bearberry and valerian).

▶ Pour cold water over the dried herb and let steep for eight to ten hours, stirring occasionally. Strain, then heat the tea to just below the boiling point.

● *Decoction* is a method primarily used for the woody parts of an herb, such as roots and bark.

▶ Using a ceramic pot, pour cold water over the herb. Heat and let simmer on low heat for five minutes. Steep for five minutes, then strain.

Preparations and Supplements

Supplements, such as tablets and capsules, and other commercially available preparations, such as syrups, tinctures, and ointments, offer the advantage of providing standardized, i.e. precisely specified, amounts of an herb's active ingredients. Syrups (e.g., fennel, ribwort, or thyme syrup) that contain at least fifty percent sugar keep well and are suitable for children. Tinctures, unlike tablets or capsules, are easy to swallow, but they contain alcohol and are therefore not recommended for children, alcoholics, and people with liver disease.

Brush your teeth after taking preparations containing sugar

Important: Always swallow tablets and capsules with sufficient liquid to reduce the risk of choking.

Important!

Fresh Juice

Certain vitamins and flavors are easily destroyed and are best obtained from fresh juices. In recent years, fresh-pressed herbal juices have become more popular again. Many people used them for juice cures in the spring.

Recipe

▶ Coarsely chop fresh herbs, let them steep in cold water for a few minutes, then put them through a juicer. You can also chop herbs in a blender, add some water, and strain them through a thin cloth. Stinging nettle, dandelion, watercress, sorrel, ribwort, and other spring herbs are all suitable for juicing, as are radishes, carrots, and celery root.

Tinctures

Tinctures are made by steeping fresh or dried herbs in alcohol. Since alcohol is a good solvent, many of the active ingredients found in fresh herbs are preserved in tinctures. These can be used in diluted form either externally for compresses and baths, or internally in herbal teas, poured over sugar cubes, or mixed with honey.

Recipe

▶ Pour 70 percent alcohol over two handfuls (a little less than a half-pound) of herb. Let the mixture steep for two weeks in a tightly closed jar kept in a dark place. Shake every two to three days. Strain through a thin cloth and fill the finished tincture into a small, brown glass bottle.

Herbal Vinegar

Herbal vinegars allow you to flavor dishes to taste, plus they serve as a digestive aid.

Recipe

▶ Put a few herbs, leaves and stems, into a bottle. Dill, tarragon, or thyme are only a few of many choices. Add organic pear, plum, or apple vinegar to the top. Allow the mixture to steep in a warm, bright room for two weeks. There is no need to remove the herbs from the finished vinegar.

Medicinal Oils

Medicinal oils can either be used internally or externally.

Recipe

▶ Crush two handfuls of buds or freshly opened flowers with a mortar and pestle. Fill a large jar with a screw-on lid or a clear bottle one-third full of the crushed herb. Add olive oil to the top. Close the jar tightly and store it in a warm place, if possible in direct sun, for about four weeks. Shake it every two to three days. Strain through a thin cloth and pour the finished oil into small, dark glass bottles.

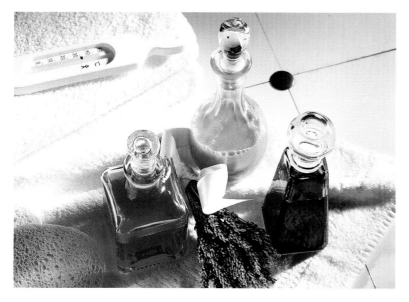

Depending on the ingredients you use, herbal baths can be either relaxing or stimulating

Herbal Baths

Herbs rich in volatile oils can transform an ordinary bath into a relaxing experience for body and soul. Herbal baths improve blood circulation and relieve tension.

▶ Place herbs on a piece of thin cotton fabric. Tie the fabric into a pouch and hang it directly under the faucet while you let the water run into the bathtub. Soak in the tub for twenty minutes, then dry yourself off and rest in a warm bed for thirty minutes. Use stimulating herbs (such as rosemary) in the morning, calming ones (such as hops or lemon balm) at night.

Recipe

Tea Mixtures

You can prepare your own tea mixtures from herbs bought in bulk from a health food or natural food store. There are various standard mixtures for urinary bladder and kidney ailments, gallbladder problems, colds, sore throats, coughs, and indigestion. Other mixtures are known for their sedative effect. A good tea mixture is made up of a maximum of four to seven different herbs. If you add more, you lose the specific effects of each herb. Mixtures generally consist of a main or dominant herb, with other herbs added in to promote the healing action. Teas sometimes include other natural ingredients, such as marigold flowers, hollyhock blossoms, or rose hip skins, to enhance flavor and appearance.

▶ Pour a cup of boiling water over one to two teaspoons of tea mixture. Let steep for five to ten minutes.

Recipe .

Aloe Vera

Herbal Gel for the Skin

Nefertiti and Cleopatra are said to have owed their irresistible beauty in large part to aloe vera. Yet for many centuries, people have used this remarkable plant for more than a beauty aid. The old herbal books of the Greeks, Romans, and Chinese praised aloe vera for its healing properties, and recommended it as a pain reliever and as a treatment for burns, hemorrhoids, and wounds. Alexander the Great had his wounded soldiers treated with aloe. The Mayas, several Native American tribes, and Tibetan monks developed various remedies using aloe. Today, aloe serves as an ornamental and a medicinal plant in many countries throughout the world. In the Caribbean, aloe juice still is a common folk remedy.

How to Recognize Aloe Vera

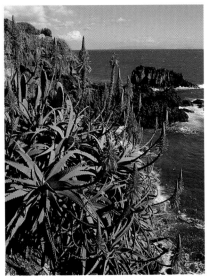

Aloe vera growing wild on Madeira

There are over 200 species of aloe vera. Although most of them resemble cacti, they actually belong to the lily family. Some aloe species look like agaves. We only use the genuine aloe, *Aloe vera barbadensis*, for medicinal purposes. This species is common in East and South Africa, as well as in the more arid areas of Europe, the Americas, and in parts of India and Australia. The aloe vera plant has a short stem that carries a rosette of leaves measuring about twenty inches in length and two inches in width. The leaves have purple marginal spines and exude a watery, very bitter gel when they are cut. Aloe plants growing in their native habitat carry tall spikes of mostly orange-colored flowers.

Cultivating and Harvesting Aloe Vera

Aloe requires well-drained soil lightly fertilized in spring and summer

In areas that tend to get frost in the winter, aloe vera must be grown in greenhouses or indoors in sunrooms in order to produce gel that contains adequate amounts of active ingredients for medicinal use. Aloe plants are easy to care for. They require little water during the winter. In the summer, they can be transplanted from their pots to a sunny spot in the garden. However, they need to be repotted and taken indoors again before the first frost. Aloe self-propagates by means of shoots. For external use, harvest the lower, older leaves.

Why Aloe Is So Valuable

The thickened sap of the leaves is used for healing. Aloe contains a number of active ingredients. Among them are mucilage, B vitamins, minerals, the bitter alloin, essential amino acids, and polysaccharides (long-chain sugar molecules). The plant's effectiveness as an immune system booster is due to a substance called acemannan. Acemannan is a kind of cell defense that the human body is able to manufacture until it reaches puberty. After that, the substance needs to be obtained from food. By strengthening the immune system, acemannan helps the body fight all kinds of infections. Aloe is also effective in treating damage caused by radiation. The mucilage contained in its leaves is used to relieve pain, stem inflammations, and promote healing of wounds.

A fortifier for the immune system, a digestive aid, and a remedy for skin disorders

Unwanted Side Effects

Fresh juice from cut aloe leaves should not be taken internally. It acts as a very strong laxative and can cause severe potassium and magnesium deficiencies and lead to constipation or irregular heartbeat (cardiac arrhythmia).

How to Use Aloe Vera

In Africa, Australia, and the Caribbean the juice of cut aloe leaves is collected in pots, thickened over a fire or in a double boiler, and usually made into a powder. This powder is then used to prepare gel for external use, or juice, tincture, tablets, capsules, oil, ointments, or suppositories for internal applications. Alloin, which is responsible for aloe's laxative effect, is removed from many preparations.

Preparations that contain no alloin are suitable for internal use

Fresh Leaves

Fresh aloe gel produces the best results. Break off a lower leaf and cut off its spines. Cut the leaf down the middle, and either place half of it directly onto the affected area of the skin, or remove and apply the gel from the inside of the leaf. Fresh leaves can be kept in the refrigerator for a few days.

Gel

This kind of preparation is commercially available and intended for external use only.

Juice Cure

Recipe

▶ Mix 1 to 1 3/4 ounces of commercially available aloe vera juice with 1 3/4 ounces of fruit juice (e.g., pineapple or orange) or wheat grass juice, according to taste and desired effect. Take three times a day for about three weeks.

Facial Mask

Simply apply a thick layer of aloe vera gel to your face and allow it to dry. If the skin feels too tight, mix in some almond, jojoba, or other oil to serve as a base for the mask.

You can also add aloe gel to any commercially available mask or prepare your own. The following recipe is for a facial mask you can make yourself for any type of skin.

Recipe

▶ *Here's what you need:*
1 tablespoon of aloe vera gel, 2 tablespoons of low fat yogurt
▶ *Here's how it's done:*
Mix the aloe vera gel with the yogurt and apply the mixture to your face and throat. Leave on for 20 minutes, then rinse off with luke-warm water.

When to Use Aloe Vera

Aloe is an ideal herb for skin care. It also promotes healing of wounds and reduces scarring. A diet that includes aloe vera juice can also fortify your immune system.

Main Applications at a Glance

Ailments:	Suggested Applications:
Acne	Apply gel; use a mask made with gel
Immune deficiency	Drink made with aloe vera juice
Scars	Massage aloe vera gel or cream into the affected area
Sunburn	Apply aloe vera gel or mucilage from a fresh aloe leaf
Wounds	Apply aloe vera gel or mucilage from a fresh aloe leaf

Skin Care

Aloe vera penetrates into and affects the deep layers of the skin. Its active ingredients accelerate cell regeneration, prevent dryness, and give the skin a smoother, softer appearance. Aloe vera protects the skin from intense sun and soothes sunburn. That's why it's used as an ingredient in many sunscreens.

▶ *Sunburn:*
After the skin has cooled off, keep applying aloe vera gel until the redness has subsided. Or cut off a fresh aloe leaf and allow the gel to drip onto the sunburned areas.

▶ *Wounds:*
When applied to wounds, aloe vera gel (or fresh juice from a cut leaf) speeds up the healing process and reduces the risk of scarring.

▶ *Scars:*
Massage scars regularly with aloe vera gel or cream.

▶ *Acne:*
Apply aloe vera gel mornings and evenings, and treat your skin with a facial mask of aloe vera gel once or twice a week.

Immune System Disorders

Recurring bacterial, viral or fungal infections often result in colds, urinary bladder infections, and many other ailments. Since aloe vera strengthens the immune system, it is an effective prophylactic agent against various infectious diseases. The herb is even said to significantly enhance the body's ability to fight tumor cells. Aloe vera accelerates the regeneration of every kind of cell found in the body and helps repair the damage caused by environmental toxins and radiation.

▶ *Immune deficiency, allergies:*
Drink alloin-free aloe vera juice over a period of three weeks. A mixture of equal parts of aloe and wheat grass juice is ideal.

▶ *For general prevention of illness:*
Drink aloe vera juice in the spring and in the fall.

Applications

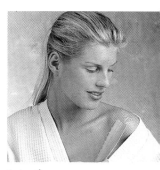

Juice from a freshly cut aloe vera leaf is very soothing to sunburned skin

Applications

Black Cumin

An Ancient Spice and Remedy

Black cumin has a long history. In Europe, it was used for centuries as a spice. The plant was also valued and widely used as a tonic and as a remedy for infections, snake bites, and rabies. It was given to women to increase lactation. The herb gradually fell into disuse during the 18th century and is only rarely cultivated in the Western world today.

In Egypt and other Middle Eastern countries, however, black cumin has been an everyday spice and remedy for more than 3000 years. It is still used there as a beauty aid for skin, hair and nails, and as a remedy to treat colds, fevers, and headaches. It also serves as a treatment for impotence and women's ailments. "Black cumin cures everything except death," is a statement attributed to the prophet Mohammed.

In European folk medicine, black cumin seeds were long used to relieve digestive ailments. The herb was also known for its wound healing properties and its ability to relieve cramps. After being nearly forgotten for almost two hundred years, reports of amazing therapeutic results obtained with black cumin have sparked renewed interest in the herb.

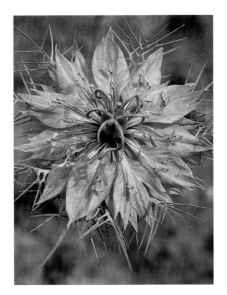

Black cumin blooms between July and September

How to Recognize Black Cumin

Genuine black cumin (*Nigella sativa*), has several other common names, among them fennel flower, nutmeg flower, or black caraway. It is not related to either caraway, the common spice, or to Indian cumin. The plant is native to the Middle East, India, and Southern Europe. Most of the black cumin seed available is imported from Egypt, since Egyptian black cumin is considered to be of exceptional quality.

The herbaceous plant, which can reach a height of about twenty inches, has hairy stems, either single or branched, with feathery, three-lobed leaves. Black cumin blooms between July and September. Its flowers are white, with petals that turn slightly green or bluish at the tips. Black seeds measuring about three millimeters in length, with three longitudinal ridges, grow inside capsules that resemble the fruits of the poppy plant.

In the Western world, black cumin is rarely seen in gardens or in the wild

Some members of the black cumin family have no medicinal properties or are even poisonous. One of them is Love-in-a-Mist (*Nigella damascena*), also known as Turkish cumin. This species is often grown here as an ornamental plant, as is the poisonous *Nigella garidella*.

How to Cultivate and Harvest Black Cumin

Black cumin grows well in warm and temperate climates and can easily be cultivated in the garden. Plant the ripe black seeds in late summer. After a year, you can harvest the aerial parts, including the light-brown seed capsules, of your cumin plants. Dry both the herb and the seeds well. Since black cumin is an annual, the plant dies in the fall.

What Makes Black Cumin So Valuable

Black cumin's amazing medicinal properties are due to the synergy of several biochemically active ingredients. Aside from very high amounts of unsaturated fatty acids, the plant contains volatile oils, tannins, and bitters. The fatty acids are said to be mainly responsible for the herb's ability to regulate immune function. If the immune system tends to react too weakly or too strongly to various "invaders," black cumin can effectively correct the inappropriate response. This property makes the herb an effective prophylactic agent against colds and other infectious diseases, as well as a useful remedy for treating various allergic conditions, such as asthma, neurodermatitis, or hay fever. Another active ingredient, nigellon, alleviates bronchial spasms associated with whooping cough and asthma.

An effective remedy for infections and asthma

Black cumin seeds are also used to treat various gastrointestinal ailments, such as abdominal gas and diarrhea. Thymoquinone, another chemical constituent found in the seeds, stimulates the production of bile and is used to help prevent gallbladder colic. Black cumin also lowers blood sugar.

Undesirable Side Effects

Black cumin doesn't pose any risk of side effects. Taken in very large amounts, however, the herb can cause gastrointestinal problems. To be safe, do not exceed the recommended dosage.

! Important for Diabetics
Black cumin lowers blood sugar and should only be taken by diabetics who monitor their blood sugar levels. Consult your doctor before taking more than the average amounts of this herb.

How to Use Black Cumin

Beware of impurities

It is advisable to buy commercially available black cumin preparations only from a reputable source, such as a health food or natural food store. Products using black cumin of Egyptian origin are best. Inexpensive preparations may contain other, toxic forms of cumin. Vitamins, primarily beta-carotene and vitamin E, are added to many preparations, since black cumin seeds are a relatively poor source of these nutrients.

Tea

Recipe

▶ *This is what you need:*
Black cumin seeds, available by mail order
▶ *This is how it's done:*
Grind two teaspoons of black cumin seeds in a mortar. Pour a cup of boiling water over the paste. Let steep for ten minutes, then strain. Drink one cup twice a day.

Black Cumin as a Condiment
Use the seeds as a condiment in salads or home-made breads, or add a touch of the Orient to your coffee or tea with ground or crushed cumin seeds.

Black cumin seed oil needs to be stored in a dry, cool place

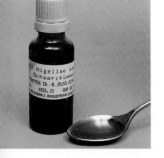

Black Cumin Seed Oil

Black cumin seed oil is available in soft gelatin capsules or as a liquid. It should be cold-pressed without chemical additives and must always be stored in a dry, cool place so it doesn't turn rancid. Liquid black cumin seed oil that has been opened can be kept for about six months.

Ozone is sometimes added to black cumin seed oil. This makes it creamy and easy to apply to the skin. Black cumin oil kills germs and gently disinfects the skin.

Important: Keep oil with added ozone away from your eyes, and do not use it for inhaling!

Inhaling, Facial Steam Baths

Recipe

▶ *This is what you need:*
Black cumin seeds, black cumin seed oil, hot water

▶ *This is how it's done:*
Measure two teaspoons of black cumin seeds and twenty drops of black cumin seed oil into a bowl. Add about two quarts of hot water. Lean over the bowl, and drape a towel over your head and the bowl. Inhale the rising steam for about ten minutes.

Dosage
For a black cumin cure, take 1.5 to 3 grams of black cumin seed oil daily for three to six months. One gram of oil is equivalent to two or three soft gelatin capsules or twenty-five drops. This is true for most commercially available preparations. For chronic conditions, take three grams of oil per day. Small children below the age of six take a third of the adult dosage, or one teaspoon of oil per day in two divided doses. Children between the ages of seven and twelve take half the adult dosage.

When to Use Black Cumin

Black cumin is primarily used to strengthen the immune system, to relieve gastrointestinal complaints, and to treat skin disorders.

Main Applications at a Glance

Ailments:	Suggested Applications:
Acne	A cure with black cumin oil, facial steam bath
Allergies	Take oil or capsules, drink tea
Asthma	Take oil or capsules, inhale
Bronchitis	Take oil or capsules, inhale
Colds, flu	A cure with black cumin oil, inhale
Fungal skin infection	Apply oil with added ozone
Gastrointestinal complaints	Take seeds, oil, or capsules, drink tea
Immune deficiency	A cure with black cumin oil
Neurodermatitis	Take oil or capsules, apply oil to skin

Immune Deficiency

People with a weakened immune system are more likely to get a cold or other infectious disease. They are also more susceptible to fungal skin infections. Added to a healthy diet and adequate outdoor exercise, black cumin can help improve your body's ability to fight off illness .

▶ *Immune deficiency:*
If you are generally susceptible to infections, take a cure with black cumin seed oil by taking one or two soft gelatin capsules daily for about six months.

▶ *Colds:*
At the first sign of a cold, such as a chill or a tickling in the throat, start taking black cumin immediately. The recommended dosage is two to three capsules three times a day. In many cases, the immune system will be sufficiently strengthened to fight off the cold. If this is not the case and you still develop a full-blown cold, the symptoms will probably be milder than usual.

Important: If the body is already weakened by a severe cold or flu, the immune system should be stimulated gently by taking only an average dosage of one capsule three times a day.

▶ *Bronchitis:*
When a cold or flu has turned into acute bronchitis, you can speed up the recovery by taking two capsules of black cumin seed oil three times a day. In addition, inhale twice a day.

Recipes

Important!

Immune Dysfunction (Allergies)

Unlike synthetic drugs, such as cortisone, natural remedies do not produce immediate results

People who are completely free of allergies are hard to find these days. Hay fever, asthma, food allergies, and neurodermatitis are all signs that the immune system is attacking harmless substances as if they were dangerous intruders. These allergic reactions by the immune system can produce only mild symptoms, such as an urge to sneeze or itchy skin, or they can lead to such serious conditions as toxic shock, a severe allergic response that can for instance be triggered by a bee sting. Treatment with black cumin can correct immune function in a very gentle manner. To accomplish this, it is necessary to take the remedy for an extended period of time.

▶ *Asthma:*
People with asthma should regularly undergo a cure with black cumin seeds. This remedy may be used in conjunction with cortisone therapy, which is often necessary for controlling asthma.

Take one or two capsules a day for three months or longer. In addition, inhale once a day.

Recipes

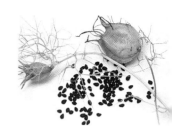

▶ *Hay fever:*
During pollen season when pollen counts are high, take two capsules three times a day. During the rest of the year, take one capsule three times daily. For acute symptoms, drink a cup of black cumin tea several times a day. When symptoms improve, you can reduce the dosage.

Gastrointestinal Complaints

The active ingredients found in black cumin seeds effectively relieve mild gastrointestinal complaints, such as feelings of fullness, heartburn, abdominal gas, diarrhea, and constipation.
▶ For acute symptoms, take two capsules three times a day. As a digestive aid, drink a cup of black cumin tea before each meal.

Recipe

Skin Disorders

Black cumin has an excellent reputation as a remedy for various skin disorders. A combination of internal and external uses is recommended in these cases. Even healthy skin can benefit from the active ingredients found in black cumin. Tired, stressed skin is made to look healthier and feels more supple. Hair and nails become shiny and strong.

!p
> **Preheat the Oil**
> Before applying undiluted oil to small areas of skin, preheat it slightly by placing the bottle into a pot with warm water. The oil will become thinner and can be better absorbed into the skin.

▶ *Acne:*
Take a cure with black cumin oil on a regular basis. Take one or two capsules three times a day for three to six months. In addition, treat yourself to several facial steam baths per week if you can.
▶ *Neurodermatitis, eczema:*
Take two to three capsules a day over a period of several months, until there is a noticeable improvement. As an added external treatment, apply undiluted black cumin oil to the affected areas several times a day.
▶ *Fungal skin infections:*
Apply ozonized black cumin oil to the affected areas three times a day. In addition, take black cumin seed oil internally in liquid or capsule form. Use the normal dosage.

Recipes

Calendula

An Herb for Treating Wounds

First mentioned by Saint Hildegard of Bingen in the 12th century as a remedy for digestive problems, eczema, and animal bites, calendula became fashionable as a cure for cancer in the 19th century. Today, the plant is used primarily to promote wound healing. Its common name is pot marigold. The Latin name Calendula is usually used when referring to the herb in a medicinal context.

How to Recognize the Pot Marigold

The pot marigold (*Calendula officinalis*) is an annual and grows to a height of about twenty-four inches. The entire plant, except for the flowers, is covered with fine hairs. Ridged stems, branched in the upper parts, bear oblong leaves. The plant produces very beautiful, yellow-orange flowers that bloom from June to November. Originally native to southeastern Europe, the pot marigold is now widely cultivated all over the world.

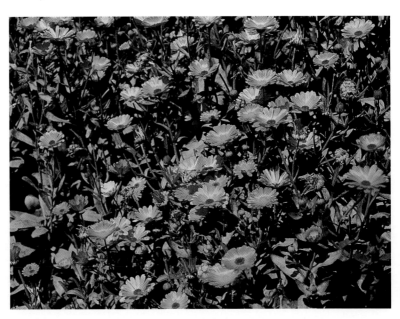

Pot marigolds spread very quickly and grow in great profusion

How to Cultivate and Harvest Pot Marigolds

The pot marigold grows in almost any soil, but it does best in sunny locations. Seeds are sown directly in the garden as early as

March. The growing seedlings need to be thinned to about a foot between individual plants. Pot marigolds usually self-propagate. The flowers which are slightly resinous, are picked in sunny, dry weather as soon as they are fully open. Carefully remove the petals, one by one, and dry them in a shady, well ventilated place.

What Makes Calendula So Effective

The plant's main active ingredients are volatile oils, flavonoids, bitters, and saponins. They promote the growth of new tissue and are responsible for the herb's anti-inflammatory, antibiotic, and wound healing properties. Calendula is an effective remedy for treating slow-healing or infected wounds, damaged skin or mucous membranes, burns, and frostbite. Calendula ointment is also used in skin care to protect and moisturize sensitive, stressed, or mature skin.

Calendula promotes healing of injuries

How to Use Calendula

Calendula tea taken internally has no clinically proven health benefits, but the yellow-orange flowers are often added to tea mixtures because of their beautiful colors.

Ointment

The best known and most common application of calendula is in the form of a salve. Calendula ointment can be applied directly to the affected skin or used in conjunction with a pack or wrap applied to the affected area. Many preparations, such as echinacea, use calendula in combination with vitamins and other herbs.

Strong Tea

You can use strong calendula tea for gargling or rinsing or to saturate a cloth or towel for a compress or wrap.
▶ Pour a cup of hot water over one to two teaspoons of dried calendula flowers. Let steep for ten minutes, then strain.

Recipe

When to Use Calendula

Deep cuts, open lacerations, or punctures involving fairly large foreign objects in the wound must be treated by a doctor. Boils on the face, head, or neck also need to be checked by a doctor.

✚ See a doctor

Main Applications at a Glance

Ailments:	Suggested Applications:
Acne	Warm facial compress using tea
Bedsores (decubitus)	Rub in calendula ointment
Boils	Dab on ointment; apply warm compresses
Eczema	Warm compresses; rub in ointment
Infected wounds	Dab on ointment; apply warm wraps or compresses
Inflammations of mouth or throat	Gargle or rinse with tea
Lacerations or contusions	Warm wraps; compresses with tea or ointment
Slow-healing wounds	Warm wraps, compresses with tea or ointment
Sunburn, mild burns	Warm compresses with strong tea
Ulcers	Warm wraps, compresses with tea or ointment

Skin and Mucous Membranes

With open wounds, always be sure that your tetanus shot is up to date

Moist packs or compresses with strong calendula tea are excellent for treating wounds and various sores, such as on the lower legs. Always make sure that the cotton or gauze you apply to a wound that is already infected, or at risk of infection, is as clean and germ-free as possible. When cleaning a wound with calendula tea, be careful not to disturb freshly formed scabs. Allow them to heal and fall off naturally to prevent prevent scarring.

Recipes

▶ *Minor infected wounds, boils:*
Dab the infected area with calendula ointment several times a day, and dress the wound with a sterile bandage if necessary. You can also apply a warm pack or compress (see pages 161 and 162) with calendula tea. Use adhesive tape to keep the bandage in place.

▶ *Acne:*
Apply a warm facial compress (see page 162) with strong calendula tea twice a week.

▶ *Slow-healing wounds, sores:*
Apply warm packs or compresses (see pages 161 and 162) with calendula tea or ointment several times a day.

▶ *Minor lacerations, contusions, or burns:*
Apply warm compresses with calendula tea several times a day.

▶ *Eczema:*
Apply calendula ointment to the affected area several times a day. For larger affected areas, apply warm packs with calendula tea. In addition, you can wash your entire body with apple cider vinegar (see page 169) and take regular chamomile baths (see page 163).

▶ *Bedsores:*
Massage areas at risk of developing bedsores with calendula ointment several times a day. Apply calendula ointment to existing bedsores as often as possible.

▶ *Infections of the mouth or throat:*
Rinse the mouth or gargle with warm calendula tea several times a day.

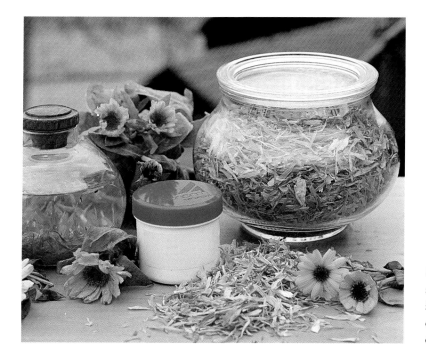

Calendula is used primarily in the form of an ointment or a tea

Chamomile

A Gentle, Versatile Herb

Chamomile is one of the most popular and versatile herbs. It has served countless people throughout their entire lives, from infancy to old age, as a remedy for pain, cramps, and injuries. That's been the case for thousands of years; in antiquity chamomile was used much as it is today. In ancient Egypt, it was worshipped as the flower of the sun good Ra. Even our stone-age ancestors seem to have known of its medicinal properties. Chamomile is one of the most widely studied herbs we have.

How to Recognize Chamomile

The hardy, unassuming chamomile (*Chamomilla recutita*, *Matricaria chamomilla*) is found throughout Europe, North America, and Australia. It often grows on uncultivated land, in overgrown dumps, and along roadsides. The German chamomile, which

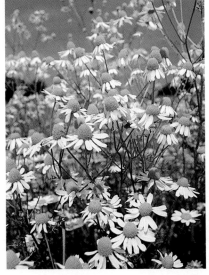

is the only member of the family used for medicinal purposes, grows about a foot and a half high and has a round, branching stem with very finely cut, yellowish-green leaves. Each shoot carries a single terminal flower head consisting of a cone shaped disc with countless tubular florets surrounded by a ring of elongated white petals. Its hollow disc and characteristic aromatic scent distinguish German chamomile from ox-eye chamomile, false chamomile, and Roman chamomile. The latter is the only other variety that contains as many volatile oils as true chamomile. It grows to about eight to twelve inches high, and has exceptionally beautiful, solid white blossoms and downy stems. It is rarely found in the wild.

Growing and Harvesting Chamomile

Chamomile blooms from May to August

German chamomile is a hardy plant that is easy to care for. All it requires is a small, sunny area in your garden. The plant even promotes the growth of other plants in its vicinity and repels pests. Chamomile can also be grown on a deck or a porch. As early as February you can plant the tiny seeds, possibly mixed with sand for easier handling, indoors in small containers. When the seedlings are about two inches tall, they are ready to be transplanted into larger containers or pots. Space the individual plants about four inches apart. Chamomile needs a sunny location, but it should not be in full sun. Organic fertilizers are appropriate.

The herb's curative power is found only in the flowers. These should be picked on sunny days, when the white petals have started to droop. Dry the flowers well in a warm but shady and well ventilated location. Since it tends to attract moisture, the dried herb must be stored in tightly closed containers in a dark place.

Chamomile also thrives without fertilizers

What Makes Chamomile So Valuable

Chamomile's therapeutic value for cramps, plus its effectiveness in treating slow-healing wounds and inflamed skin and mucous membranes, is undisputed. The herb has also traditionally been used for its pain-relieving and calming properties. Chamomile's versatility as a remedy is due to the combined effect of several active ingredients. Volatile oils are mainly responsible for the herb's anti-inflammatory effect. Flavonoids, found in considerable amounts in the flowers, also reduce inflammation and relieve cramps. Chamomile blossoms are rich in mucilage, which reduces irritation in the mucous lining of the stomach and intestines.

Unwanted Side Effects

Chamomile is very harmless, and it causes virtually no unwanted side effects. Just the same, drinking chamomile tea on a daily basis for years is not recommended. Do not use chamomile externally to treat eye inflammation.

Allergic reactions to German chamomile are very rare. It appears that several cases reported over the last few years were attributable to contamination from ox-eye chamomile.

Commercially available preparations are usually free of impurities

How to Use Chamomile

Tea

Infusion with hot water is a good way to obtain the herb's mucilage, certain kinds of flavonoids, and a small portion of its volatile oils.

▶ Pour a cup of hot water over a heaping teaspoon of dried herb. Cover and let steep for five to ten minutes, then strain. Drink the tea as warm as possible and while it is still fresh.

Recipe

Chamomile Extract

When treating more severe symptoms, this preparation is generally preferable to tea. Extracts contain considerably larger amounts of volatile oils, which are removed from the plant with alcohol. Like tea, extracts are commercially available in health food and natural food stores. Choose preparations with standardized amounts of chemically active ingredients. The recommended dosage varies among the different products.

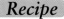 *Recipe*

▶ Dissolve a small amount of chamomile extract in warm water. Drink the mixture as a tea, or use it for gargling, inhaling, or for compresses. For correct dosage, follow the directions on the label.

Strong Tea

For gargling, rinsing, inhaling, or for packs and compresses, you need a strong tea.

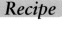 *Recipe*

▶ Pour a cup of hot water over three to five heaping teaspoons of chamomile flowers. Let steep for five to ten minutes, then strain.

Baths

▶ Tie chamomile flowers (two ounces for every three gallons of bath water) into a linen sachet. Hang the sachet under the faucet of your bathtub so that the running water can release the herb's active ingredients.

Inhaling

▶ Pour about two quarts of hot water over a handful of dried chamomile flowers placed in a bowl. Lean over the bowl and drape a towel over your head and the bowl. Inhale the rising steam for about ten minutes.

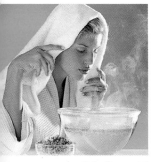

Inhaling with chamomile is helpful for colds

Chamomile Oil

Chamomile oil is recommended for external use and can be made at home.

▶ Fill a glass jar with a screw-on lid with fresh, crushed chamomile flowers. Add olive oil, close tightly, and store for three to four weeks in a sunny location. Strain the infused oil through a thin cloth. If you wish, add a few drops of high-quality volatile chamomile oil, available from health food or natural food stores, if desired. Store the oil in a tightly closed bottle.

Ointments

Chamomile ointments for external use, containing the herb's biologically active ingredients, are available commercially.

Homeopathic Remedies

The homeopathic remedy "Chamomilla" is prepared from the whole chamomile plant. It is used primarily for ailments related to a hypersensitive nervous system, such as neuralgia (sharp pain extending along a nerve or group of nerves) and certain head- or toothaches, or for abdominal cramps.

When to Use Chamomile

Chamomile is helpful for treating several types of skin conditions and hereditary ailments.

Main Applications at a Glance

Ailments:	Suggested Applications:
Colds	Drink tea, gargle, inhale
Dry skin	Rub in oil or ointment
Gastritis	Rolling cure with chamomile tea
Gastrointestinal complaints	Camomile tea, tea cure in conjunction with fasting
Gingivitis	Rinse with strong chamomile tea
Inflammation, blemished skin	Facial steam baths, compresses with oil, partial baths
Teething	Homeopathic remedy Chamomilla
Wounds	Compresses with strong chamomile tea

Gastrointestinal Complaints

Chamomile brings quick relief for various ailments of the gastrointestinal tract, such as nausea, belching, inflammation of the mucous lining of the stomach (gastritis), and abdominal gas. People often take antacids to relieve nervous indigestion. Since this condition is often brought on by emotional stress and anxiety, a gentle, calming remedy such as chamomile is a much better treatment.

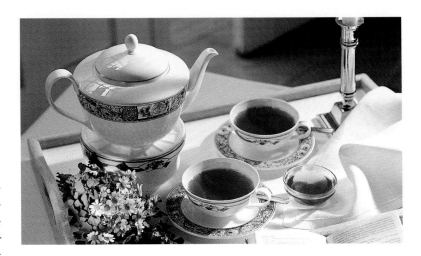

Chamomile tea with honey is an effective remedy for colds

✚ **You must see a doctor**

Recipes

Important: If symptoms persist, or if blood is present in stool or vomit, you *must* see a doctor to be checked for stomach or duodenal ulcers. In consultation with the doctor, you may be able to use chamomile tea in conjunction with conventional medical treatment.

▶ For all gastrointestinal ailments, drink three to four cups of warm chamomile tea on an empty stomach. For acute cases, fast for three days and drink tea: chamomile tea, or peppermint tea for variety, bed rest, and moist, warm packs or wraps applied to the abdomen (see page 160) are a very effective treatment. After fasting, start slowly with low salt, low fat soups made with rice, flour, or millet.

▶ *Inflammation of the mucous lining of the stomach (gastritis):* Use a procedure called a "rolling cure": slowly sip two cups of warm chamomile tea. Lie down on your back and relax. After five minutes, turn onto your left side, then onto your stomach, and finally onto your right side. Rest for 5 minutes in each position. Do this procedure in the morning and again at night, if desired.

Colds

Chamomile is known to relieve sore throats and general fatigue, often the first signs of a cold. It is also an effective remedy for nasal congestion and prevents the infection from spreading to the sinuses and bronchi.

Recipes

▶ *Sore throat:* Prepare a strong tea, using three teaspoons of chamomile flowers per cup of hot water. Use it as hot as you can stand, for gargling at least three times a day, or more frequently if needed. Drink three cups of warm tea sweetened with honey every day.

▶ *Colds, sinus, or throat infections:* Traditional facial steam baths with chamomile are an excellent treatment for these conditions.

Oral Infections

Gingivitis and other oral infections can be treated by rinsing with chamomile.

▶ Prepare a strong tea with three teaspoons of chamomile per cup of water. For acute conditions, slosh it around in your mouth for a minute at a time three times a day, or more frequently if necessary.

Recipe

Skin Conditions

Chamomile is a very effective remedy for slow-healing wounds, varicose sores, and bedsores. It is ideal for cleansing and moisturizing dry, sensitive skin.

▶ *Slow-healing wounds:*
Compresses with strong chamomile tea are usually very effective.

▶ *Dry, rough skin:*
After a shower or bath, regularly apply chamomile ointment to chapped skin. Rub or massage the entire body with home-made chamomile oil. For facial care, first moisten your hands with warm water. Pour a small amount of chamomile oil into your palms and apply it evenly to the face. It will leave your skin smooth and supple.

▶ *Blemished, sensitive skin:*
For a full body treatment, take a chamomile bath. For local inflammation confined to a smaller area of the body, apply chamomile oil compresses (see page 162). Partial baths (see pages 164–165) are recommended for skin inflammation in the genital area. Steam baths two to three times a week are very beneficial as a facial treatment. Follow the directions for inhaling.

Recipes

A Sick Child

Because it tastes good and is easy to digest, cure-all chamomile is an ideal remedy for various ailments in small children and infants.

▶ *Stomach pains, abdominal gas, and diarrhea:*
Have the child sip very warm chamomile tea. Warm stomach wraps or packs provide additional relief.

▶ *Cold or other infectious diseases:*
Dissolve one teaspoon of honey per cup of chamomile tea. Do not use honey if treating a child under one year of age. Give as a general tonic.

▶ *Teething, colic:*
Administer the homeopathic form of chamomile. Place five to ten tablets of Chamomilla onto the child's tongue three to five times a day and let them dissolve slowly.

Recipes

Chaste Tree

A Mediterranean Herb for Women

Chaste tree's role as a remedy throughout history can be gleaned from its common and Latin names. "Agnus castus" means "chaste lamb." Both names indicate that the herb was believed to inhibit sexual desire. This notion was wrong and based on an error in translation. Nevertheless, monks used the plant's spicy, peppery fruits to keep their sexual desire under control.

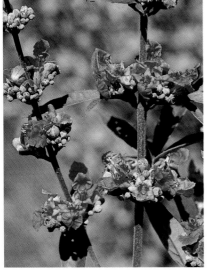

Two other common names, monk's pepper and hemp tree, point to other uses of this shrub. In Europe's southern regions, the plant's fruits were also used as a substitute for pepper. Its supple twigs were woven into baskets, hence its name "Vitex," which is derived from the Latin word for basket weaving.

Today, chaste tree is mainly used as a remedy for symptoms associated with the female menstrual cycle.

Identifying Chaste Tree

Chaste tree (*Vitex agnus castus*) commonly grows along riverbanks and the coast in Central Asia and the Mediterranean. It grows to about twelve feet in height and has lance-shaped, palmate compound leaves. They are dark-green on top and white and downy on the underside. From July until August, the shrubs carry pale purple, pink, or white flowers. Chaste tree fruits used for medicinal purposes are

Chaste tree blooms in July and August

fairly large, reddish-black berries about an inch in diameter. They taste spicy, somewhat like pepper.

How to Cultivate and Harvest Chaste Tree

Chaste tree is grown in temperate climates as an ornamental plant. The deciduous shrub can be planted either in containers or in the garden. It prefers sunny locations and rather moist soil. The ripe fruits, "monk's peppercorns," are picked in September or October. They are dried and processed into various preparations for medicinal use.

What Makes Chaste Tree So Effective

The main active ingredients found in chaste tree berries are volatile and fatty oils, flavonoids, iridoid glycosides, and bitters. These compounds act together to inhibit the production of the hormone prolactin by the pituitary gland. The female body naturally produces more prolactin during lactation, resulting in (temporary) infertility and cessation of periods—a wise provision of nature during that phase in a woman's life. Elevated prolactin levels can also be produced by stress, however, and can lead to irregular menstrual cycles, premenstrual syndrome, decreased libido, and even infertility.

Too much prolactin can lead to infertility and irregular periods

Undesirable Side Effects

Chaste tree should not be used during pregnancy or while nursing a baby. If you are taking prescription neuroleptic drugs (potent tranquilizers), talk to your doctor before taking chaste tree preparations; there may be some drug interactions. There have been rare cases of eczematous dermatitis associated with taking this herb.

Not recommended during pregnancy or while nursing

How to Use Chaste Tree

Chaste tree preparations cannot be made at home; you have to get them at health food and natural food stores. Dosage is dependent upon the amount of active ingredients in each individual product. Please read and follow the instructions on the label.

Alcohol-based Extracts

Commercially available extracts contain the active ingredients of chaste tree alone, or in combination with additional ingredients derived from other plants.

Capsules

Capsules have the advantage of containing no alcohol.

Homeopathic Remedies

These preparations are used to treat impotence in men or to stop milk production in women. They usually are mixtures of medicines containing other homeopathic remedies as well as chaste tree.

When to Use Chaste Tree

Important: If you are experiencing any of the symptoms described in this chapter, you should consult a gynecologist.

Main Applications at a Glance

Ailments:	Suggested Applications:
Irregular menstrual cycle	Take extract or capsules
Premenstrual syndrome	Take extract or capsules

Premenstrual Syndrome

Chaste tree is an effective remedy for treating the symptoms many women experience before the onset of their menstrual periods (premenstrual syndrome). These symptoms include swollen, tender breasts, headaches, emotional swings, constipation, and water retention in tissue. Roughly half of all women suffer from premenstrual syndrome at some time during their lives.

Recipe

▶ Take capsules or extract for at least four months until symptoms diminish. For proper dosage, follow the directions on the label.

Irregular Menstrual Cycle

First consult your doctor

With its gentle action on the hormonal system, chaste tree is an effective remedy for regulating a woman's menstrual cycle. In case of irregular periods, you should consult your gynecologist before taking chaste tree.

Recipe

▶ With your doctor's approval, take chaste tree capsules or extract over a period of several weeks, until your cycle returns to normal. For proper dosage, follow the instructions on the label.

Echinacea

A Great Immune System Stimulant

The purple coneflower, better known by its Latin name, Echinacea, is native to North America. It was one of the most popular herbs used by the Native Americans, who valued it primarily as a treatment for slow-healing wounds. In addition, Echinacea served as a remedy for pain, poisoning, cramps, and breast cancer, and it was used to increase the body's resistance to all kinds of infections.

Echinacea found its way into conventional medicine in the 18th century. Knowledge of its curative powers, at first in homeopathic applications, spread at the start of the 20th century. After several decades of popularity, Echinacea faded from view in the 1930s when the first sulfa drugs appeared on the market. In herbal medicine, Echinacea continues to be widely used as an immune system stimulant.

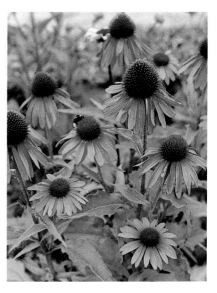

Identifying Echinacea

In its native North American habitat, the narrow-leaved Echinacea (*Echinacea angustifolia*) and the pale-flowered Echinacea (*Echinacea pallida*) are found in dry soil such as sandy riverbanks, on prairies, and in dry forests. The purple coneflower (*Echinacea purpurea*) is the species commonly cultivated for medicinal use. The plant can be recognized by its cone-shaped, purple flowers and its oblong, smooth-edged leaves. Both stems and leaves are covered with fine hairs. Echinacea blooms from July to September. *Echinacea angustifolia* grows to a height of about eighteen inches, while *Echinacea purpurea* reaches twice that height.

The cone-shaped flowers of Echinacea gave the plant its common name

How to Cultivate and Grow Echinacea

Most climates in the United States are suitable for growing Echinacea outdoors, either in the garden or in pots on a deck or a porch. Among the various species, *Echinacea purpurea* is the best choice. It is not only rich in biochemically active ingredients, but also makes a pretty ornamental plant in the garden or on the balcony. *Echinacea pallida* is also well suited to cultivation.

Echinacea purpurea is a hardy herbaceous perennial that needs little care: it loves sunny locations, but also tolerates partial shade.

Echinacea grows well in most gardens

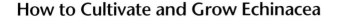

If you want to provide additional nutrients, you can enrich the soil with compost or organic fertilizer.

When the plant reaches a height of about eighteen inches, it should be supported with stakes to keep the stalks from bending or breaking. The fresh Echinacea plants are best picked right after they come into bloom, then hung up to dry in a shady, dark place. Fresh roots, however, are not harvested until the fall, when they are cleaned, coarsely chopped, and dried separately. The dried herb can be preserved in alcohol or mixed with a base to make an ointment.

What Makes Echinacea So Valuable

The most significant active ingredient found in all Echinacea species is echinacin. But there are many other substances that contribute to the herb's overall effectiveness: volatile oils, flavonoids, resins, bitters, and phytosterols. *Echinacea purpurea* also contains alkaloids and vitamin C.

Echinacea is known primarily for its effect on the immune system. The herb increases the number of white corpuscles in the blood and stimulates the activity of natural killer cells. All systems of the body involved in the production of new blood cells are strengthened by Echinacea. Treatment with Echinacea is even said to be as effective as antibiotic therapy in many cases. Studies have shown that the herb relieves coughing in children with pertussis (whooping cough) within two weeks, just as with antibiotics. In untreated patients, the symptom lasted for four to eight weeks. In addition, children treated with Echinacea did not experience the coughing spasms typically associated with the disease.

Echinacea increases the concentration of stress hormones in the blood necessary to fight illness

Used externally, echinacoside, another active ingredient found in the roots of *E. angustifolia,* is effective in protecting the body against bacteria, viruses, and fungi. While this chemical compound doesn't kill these organisms, it keeps them from entering the body. It also inhibits the growth of fungi. Echinacoside stimulates the production of fibroblasts, the repair material of tissue, thereby limiting swelling and infection.

Undesirable Side Effects

Echinacea, when applied externally, keeps germs from entering the body

People with allergies to plants of the daisy family can experience nausea or diarrhea when taking Echinacea. When used externally, the herb can cause burning, itching, or rashes. In such cases, discontinue treatment.

Echinacea preparation should be avoided by people diagnosed with AIDS and HIV-infections, multiple sclerosis, tuberculosis, leukemia, various collagen diseases (lupus, scleroderma, rheumatoid arthritis), and other auto-immune disorders.

Important: Echinacea should not be taken for more than eight weeks at a time. Long-term treatment beyond eight weeks poses the risk of an adverse reaction by the immune system. Any treatment with Echinacea of severely ill people should be conducted under the supervision of a medical doctor.

Important!

How to Use Echinacea

Buy Echinacea preparations only from a reputable source. Many products are adulterated with other herbs. The normal dose for adults is forty drops of alcohol-based tincture, the most frequently encountered form, taken three times a day. Small children should receive five drops, older children ten drops dissolved in liquid up to five times a day. Tablets, which are free of alcohol, are also available.

Beware of adulterated products

Intensive Treatment

When treating infections with Echinacea, starting with a high initial dose, followed by smaller doses at short intervals during the first day, has produced good results. Dosage on the first day:
● Adults: 40 drops initially, then 20 drops every one to two hours (starting on the second day, 40 drops three times daily)
● Older children: 20 drops initially, then ten drops every one to two hours
● Small children: 10 drops initially, then 5 drops every one to two hours

> **! Please Note**
> Do not use Echinacea preparations (including ointment!)
> in children younger than one year. Children with
> allergies should not be treated with Echinacea until
> age three.

Tincture, Tablets, Capsules, and Alcohol-free Glycerite

● Alcohol-based Echinacea tinctures contain juice squeezed from Echinacea roots. They are least allergenic because they contain virtually no proteins, the allergens to which the body reacts.

● Tablets, capsules, chewable tablets, and glycerite can be used by people who wish to avoid alcohol.
● For injections, physicians and health practitioners in Europe use special Echinacea preparations made from the above-ground parts of the plant.

Each patient must be checked for allergies before injections are administered.

Lozenges, Gargling Solutions, Mouthwashes

Lozenges, gargling solutions, and mouthwashes are recommended for infections of the upper respiratory tract, since they start their therapeutic action right in the throat.

Tea, Paste for Poultices

Recipe

▶ Pour a cup of boiling water over two teaspoons of dried herb, cover and let steep for ten minutes, then strain.
▶ Finely chop two fresh or dried roots, or an entire plant. Grind the dried herb with a mortar and pestle, add some water, and puree it in a blender. When using fresh herb, puree directly, without crushing first.

Ointment, Lipstick, Soap

Echinacea ointment is used for treating the skin. Echinacea lipstick helps heal cracked, sore lips. Blemished skin or acne can be washed with Echinacea soap.

Homeopathic Preparations

Homeopathic practitioners use Echinacea mainly for treating the same ailments that are commonly treated with herbal Echinacea preparations.

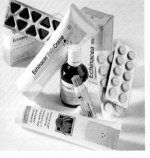

An abundance of different Echinacea preparations are available on the market

When to Use Echinacea

Echinacea serves mainly as a treatment for all kinds of infections. It can also be used in conjunction with antibiotics to strengthen the immune system.

Important!

Important: Before taking Echinacea supplements, discuss using the herb and the appropriate dosage with your doctor. Continue taking Echinacea for an additional one to two weeks after completion of antibiotic treatment.

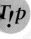 **For Your Travel First Aid Kit**
Take Echinacea along on your travels: ointment helps with
insect bites and minor skin injuries. Tinctures, capsules, and
tablets help ward off infections. For wraps or rinses, you can
crush Echinacea tablets and dissolve them in boiled water.

Immune Deficiency

During periods of increased risk of infection (using air condition-
ing, contact with many people, immune deficiency, hospital stay,
traveling abroad) or before an important event when you want to
make sure to avoid catching a cold, take an Echinacea cure.

▶ Take 40 drops in some water three times a day after meals for
three weeks. Repeat the cure after three weeks if desired.

Recipe

Eye Infections

Echinacea is also an effective remedy for eye infections, such as
conjunctivitis, sties, or blepharitis (infection of the eyelid).

▶ Apply a poultice with freshly prepared Echinacea paste or ointment to the closed eye and leave it on for about fifteen minutes.
Repeat if needed.

Recipe

◀Main Applications at a Glance

Ailments:	Suggested Applications:
Cold, flu	Take tincture, starting with a high initial dose
Cold sores	Apply ointment or tincture
Fungal skin infection	Apply ointment, take tincture
Immune deficiency	Take tincture
Infected wounds	Apply ointment; poultice with paste or diluted tincture
Infections of the mouth or throat	Gargle with diluted tincture
Shingles	Wrap with paste or diluted tincture; take tincture internally
Urinary bladder infection	Take drops, starting with a high initial dose
Vaginal yeast infection	Take tincture

Colds

In taking Echinacea for a cold, it's important to choose the right type of plant. Preparations made with *Echinacea purpurea* are very effective for colds, but ones that contain *Echinacea angustifolia* hardly produce any results at all.

Recipe

▶ At the first signs of a cold, start with a high initial dosage on the first day, then reduce to the normal dosage and continue taking until the symptoms are gone.

Urinary Tract Infections

Infections of the urinary tract, also called urinary bladder infections, or irritable bladder symptoms can also be successfully treated with Echinacea.

Recipe

▶ Start with a high dosage on the first day, then cut back to the normal dosage. In addition, alternate between drinking Echinacea tea, kidney and bladder tea, and apple cider vinegar-honey drink (see page 18).

Skin and Mucous Membranes

Skin infections caused by viruses, bacteria or fungi, as well as slow-healing wounds respond very well to Echinacea treatment. Preparations with *Echinacea purpurea* are very effective in treating herpes, but those that contain *Echinacea angustifolia* are of little use.

Recipes

▶ *Cold sores, shingles:*
At the first signs of infection, apply some ointment to the affected area. To relieve shingles, apply a poultice of Echinacea paste or a wrap with diluted tincture (see page 160). In addition, take tincture internally.
▶ *Infected or slow-healing wounds:*
Apply Echinacea ointment to the wound, or apply a poultice of Echinacea paste or a compress with diluted tincture (see page 161).
▶ *Infections of the mouth or throat:*
Prepare a gargling solution with two parts water and one part Echinacea tincture. Gargle three times a day until the infection is gone.
▶ *Vaginal yeast infection:*
In addition to standard treatment for yeast infections prescribed by your doctor, take Echinacea tincture for eight weeks. This will considerably reduce the likelihood of recurring infection.

Evening Primrose

A Medicinal as well as a Culinary Herb

Evening primrose is native to North America. Native Americans valued it as a cure-all and used the various species of the plant to treat infections, female disorders, obesity, snake bites, and even laziness. In the early 17th century the herb was finally introduced to Europe, where it spread all throughout the continent. Farmers soon discovered its value as a nutritious vegetable: its reddish roots are long and fleshy. Only recently, scientific studies have confirmed the healing properties of evening primrose oil on the skin and its regulatory action on elevated lipid levels in the blood.

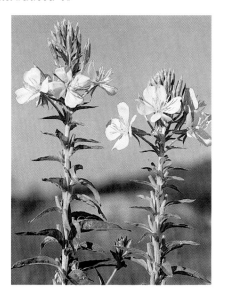

How to Recognize Evening Primrose

Evening primrose (*Oenothera biennis*) is often cultivated in gardens, but it also grows wild on vacant land, railroad embankments, and along rivers. During its first year, the biennial plant produces only an inconspicuous basal rosette of leaves. During the second year, it grows a stalk up to three feet in height with a long terminal spike of yellow flowers. The plant is pollinated during the night by moths; that's the reason for its common name. Evening primrose blooms between June and October. Its fruit capsules contain seeds that provide the oil valued for its medicinal properties.

Evening primrose flowers open in the evening and fade during the day

How to Cultivate and Harvest Evening Primrose

Evening primrose thrives in sunny locations and in sandy soil. Its ripe seeds are either cold-pressed to preserve most of their valuable active ingredients, or the oil is extracted by a specific process using carbon dioxide. Vitamin E is usually added to make the oil less perishable. The roots of the plant are dug in the spring or the fall.

What Makes Evening Primrose So Valuable

Evening primrose contains tannins, flavonoids, and mucilage in its stems and leaves. Large amounts of tannins are mainly responsible for the plant's healing effect on wounds and for its ability to relieve gastrointestinal complaints and urinary bladder infections. The most important active ingredient, however, is found in the oil contained in its seeds. This oil is very rich in rare and valuable gamma-linoleic acids, unsaturated fatty acids needed by the body for beautiful, well-nourished, healthy skin that feels soft and supple. Evening primrose oil is used in skin care to prevent signs of premature aging.

The oil also has medicinal uses. It mainly serves as a treatment for neurodermatitis and can significantly reduce the symptoms associated with this skin disorder. Evening primrose oil is also effective in relieving premenstrual syndrome and lowers cholesterol levels in the blood.

Undesirable Side Effects

Rare cases of nausea, digestive problems, and headaches have been reported. Gastrointestinal problems can be avoided by taking the capsules after eating. With a doctor's approval, evening primrose oil can be taken during pregnancy (only after the first trimester) and while nursing.

How to Use Evening Primrose

All the major evening primrose preparations use oil from the plant's seeds. They must be made professionally, rather than at home.

Capsules, Creams

Evening primrose oil usually comes in 500-milligram soft gelatin capsules. If you do not like to swallow capsules, you can cut them open, squeeze out the oil, and drink it with some fluid. Regular use for at least eight weeks is usually necessary for noticeable improvement. After that, you can cut down the dosage. Skin care creams containing evening primrose oil are now also commercially available.

When to Use Evening Primrose

Evening primrose oil is used primarily for treating the skin. It is very effective in relieving the symptoms of neurodermatitis.

Main Applications at a Glance

Ailments:	Suggested Applications:
Dry skin	Take capsules, rub in diluted oil
Elevated cholesterol levels	Take capsules
Neurodermatitis	Take capsules, rub in full-strength oil
Premenstrual syndrome	Take capsules

Neurodermatitis, dry skin

After a few weeks of treatment with evening primrose oil, the skin of patients suffering from neurodermatitis usually feels less dry, is less scaly, and itching and irritation are reduced. Used either internally or externally, the oil is an effective remedy for excessively dry skin.

▶ Adults suffering from neurodermatitis take four to six capsules twice a day; children over the age of one take two to four capsules a day after meals. The dosage can be reduced as needed after symptoms improve.

Recipe

For dry skin, take four to six capsules twice a day after meals for eight weeks during the winter months.

Premenstrual Syndrome

If you regularly experience lower back pain, tender breasts, headaches, irritability, or depression before the onset of your period, use evening primrose oil during the second half of your menstrual cycle.

▶ Take evening primrose capsules for several months. If your symptoms are severe, increase the dosage to as many as six capsules twice a day. Once the symptoms have improved, you can cut back on the dosage.

Recipe

Elevated Cholesterol Levels

Evening primrose oil can help regulate cholesterol levels by reducing LDL (harmful cholesterol) and increasing HDL (healthy cholesterol). If your cholesterol levels are high, you should see your doctor and ask him whether self-treatment with evening primrose oil is advisable.

✚ See a doctor

▶ Take four to six capsules of evening primrose oil twice a day.

Ginkgo

A Tonic for the Brain

Almost 200 million years ago, numerous members of the ginkgo family thrived in all parts of the world. All but one of these species disappeared as other deciduous trees and firs took over their habitat. The ginkgo biloba tree is the only survivor, a kind of living fossil, that can still be found growing virtually unchanged in small parts of Eastern Asia.

Ginkgo seeds are used in traditional Chinese medicine to treat asthma, coughs, and alcoholism. Raw seeds are said to inhibit the growth of tumors, while cooked seeds act as a digestive aid. In Europe, ginkgo leaves were used to bandage wounds, and, cooked into a paste, applied as poultices to relieve frostbite. Ginkgo tea used to be a popular remedy for bronchitis, asthma, coughs, and gastrointestinal complaints. It also served as a treatment for infertility, tuberculosis, and metabolic disorders. Today, ginkgo extract is primarily used to improve blood flow to the brain.

How to Identify the Ginkgo Tree

Ginkgo trees can grow to a towering height of up to about 125 feet. They have broad crowns and long-stemmed, two-lobed leaves. The trees do not bloom until they are at least twenty to thirty years old. The fruits produced by the ginkgo tree resemble nuts. Unlike our nuts, which contain primarily fats, the kernels of the ginkgo fruit consist mainly of starches. The fleshy outer hulls of the seeds contain toxins whose function it is to protect the tree from pests. These toxins can irritate the skin.

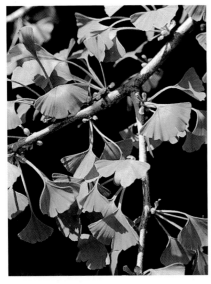

The ginkgo tree has unique, two-lobed leaves

How to Cultivate and Harvest Ginkgo

Always wear gloves when removing the hulls from ginkgo seeds

If you want to grow your own ginkgo tree, buy a small plant from a nursery. You will have to protect it from frost for the first five years. By then, your ginkgo tree may already be more than six feet tall.

Only the leaves of the ginkgo tree are used to make ginkgo extract. These leaves usually come from trees grown on plantations in Southern France, North America, China, Japan, and Korea. Ginkgo leaves are picked either individually or by the twig. Harvesting takes place in the fall when the plants contain the largest amounts of active ingredients.

What Makes Ginkgo So Valuable

Ginkgo's main active ingredients are flavone glycosides, ginkgolides, and bilabolides, which all belong to a group of chemical compounds called terpene lactones.

Ginkgo extract mainly helps maintain adequate metabolic function in the brain, even when there is a reduced supply of oxygen. It is also a free-radical scavenger and acts as a blood thinner, thereby improving circulation in the small capillaries and facilitating the elimination of metabolic waste. Because of these effects, ginkgo extract may be capable of slowing down the progress of Alzheimer's disease.

An effective remedy for increasing blood flow to brain

Undesirable Side Effects

Ginkgo extracts are very safe. Allergic reactions are very rare, and they are the only known side effect.

Ginkgo seeds are mildly toxic and should not be given to children. Even adults should consume them in small amounts.

Do not use the hulls of ginkgo seeds! They can cause severe inflammation of the gastrointestinal tract and the kidneys.

How to Use Ginkgo

While you can prepare your own tea from ginkgo leaves, extract cannot be made at home. The plant's active ingredients are extracted primarily with alcohol, utilizing a process that removes some toxic compounds and substances that could reduce the herb's therapeutic effects.

Tablets, Capsules, or Liquid Extract

A special extract prepared from green, dried ginkgo leaves is available either as a liquid, as capsules, or as tablets that are available only at health food and natural food stores. You can also get special drops that contain no alcohol.

Tea

While ginkgo tea tastes pleasant and aromatic, its effectiveness has not been clinically proven.

▶ Pour a cup of boiling water over one to two teaspoons of ginkgo leaves. Let steep for ten minutes, then drain. Add honey to taste.

Recipe

When to Use Ginkgo

✚ See a doctor *Important:* In general, people suffering from ailments typically treated with ginkgo should consult a physician.

Main Applications at a Glance

Ailments:	Suggested Applications:
Circulatory problems	Take ginkgo extract
Dizziness	Take ginkgo extract
Memory loss	Take ginkgo extract
Ringing in the ears	Take ginkgo extract

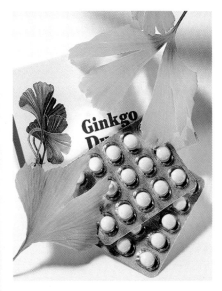

Memory loss, reduced concentration, and depression—symptoms often associated with Alzheimer's disease—can be successfully treated with ginkgo. In some cases, the progress of the disease can even be stopped. Ginkgo is said to improve the functioning of the remaining healthy nerve cells in the brains of patients and to protect them from damage. The effectiveness of ginkgo extract in treating these conditions has been clinically proven. The same, however, cannot be said for ginkgo tea.

Poor Blood Circulation in the Legs

If you regularly experience severe pain while walking due to insufficient blood flow to the legs (peripheral arterial obstruction), ginkgo in combination with physical therapy may help extend the distance you can able to walk without pain.

Ringing in the Ears, Dizziness

Ginkgo is also an effective remedy for ringing in the ears, dizziness, and headaches due to reduced blood flow to the head and brain.

✚ See a doctor immediately *Important:* See a doctor immediately if you experience sudden hearing loss or deafness. If you experience frequent dizzy spells, you should likewise see your doctor.

Ginseng

A Cure-all for Body and Soul

The ginseng plant has had a permanent place among the remedies used in Eastern Asian medicine for thousands of years. Its Chinese name is "jen-shen," which means "manlike root." Its gentle, harmonizing effect on body and soul has earned the herb the title of "prince of remedies." In 1842, ginseng was given the additional designation "Panax," meaning panacea or "cure-all."

The ginseng root is said to have been introduced to Europe by Arabian seafarers as early as the middle of the 9th century B.C. From the late 17th to the middle of the 19th century, it was popular as a tonic mainly among members of the royal courts. Enthusiasm for the herb waned, however, when cheaper, less potent American ginseng roots found their way to Europe and took the place of the expensive Asian roots.

The "manlike root" is regarded as "the prince of remedies"

Today, people in China and Korea chew ginseng root for protection against disease and environmental toxins, use the herb as a spice, and drink it as a tea. Ginseng is available in the form of pills, jellies, chewing gum, lemonade, candy, body lotions, shampoos, and even cigarettes. The herb is also regaining its popularity in Europe, where people are once more willing to pay a fair price for good quality ginseng roots.

How to Identify Ginseng

Wild ginseng (*Panax ginseng C. A. Meyer*) is native to the mountain forests of the northern, temperate zones of Asia, northeastern China, and the Korean peninsula. The plant is also cultivated for medicinal use in Japan, Thailand, Russia, Canada, and North America, but the roots grown there are of inferior quality.

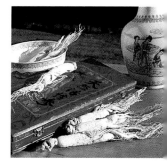

Ginseng roots have a bitter yet slightly sweet taste

Ginseng is a perennial shrub that reaches a maximum height of about three feet and produces bright red, edible berries. Slender, single stems carry saw-toothed compound leaves. The part of the plant used for its medicinal properties is the long, fleshy, light-yellow to brown root with its many long, delicate root hairs. It has an aromatic smell and tastes bitter, but also slightly sweet.

How to Cultivate and Harvest Ginseng

Cultivating ginseng is very difficult and time-consuming. The seeds take up to two years to germinate. At least another four to six years are needed for the plant to produce a root that is ready to be harvested

The quality of
ginseng varies
according
to species and
cultivation

for medicinal use. Depending on the type of processing used, the roots of Chinese or Korean ginseng are made into white or red ginseng: White ginseng root is collected after four years, dried quickly, and then processed. To obtain the highly valued red ginseng, freshly harvested roots from highland plants that are at least six years old are steamed and then dried. During this process, the roots turn reddish-orange in color and become very hard and almost translucent.

What Makes Ginseng So Valuable

The root's main active ingredients are ginsenosides, contained in very high concentrations primarily in the fine root hairs. Other ingredients include volatile oils, vitamins, minerals, and trace minerals. Maltol, a by-product of the specific process used to preserve red ginseng, is thought to play a role in the root's ability to inhibit certain processes of aging.

Ginseng stimulates the central nervous system, accelerates the transmission of nerve impulses, and increases oxygen intake by the cells. It regulates immune and metabolic functions, blood pressure, and blood sugar. Ginseng has a beneficial effect on the intestinal flora and helps the organism get rid of toxins quickly and efficiently. It also temporarily increases physical stamina and protects the body from potential damage due to radiation, infections, poisons, and from the effects of physical and psychological stress.

Undesirable Side Effects

Ginseng is very safe, even for prolonged use. It is not habit-forming, and if taken in recommended doses, there is no risk of side effects.

How to Use Ginseng

Long term use
of ginseng is safe
even for the
elderly and the
chronically ill

For best results, buy standardized products with certified amounts of ginsenosides from a reputable manufacturer. There are many products on the market that can vary widely as to the quality and quantity of ginseng they contain. Authentic ginseng is expensive. Price usually reflects ginsenoside content.

Extracts

Extracts contain high concentrations of the root's active ingredients, are readily soluble, and usually free of pesticides. They are sold in the form of capsules, powders, tablets, or concentrated liquids.

Loose Powder

This is the common form of administration in traditional Chinese medicine. The powder also comes in capsules that make it easy to get the right dosage.

Tea

Ginseng is also available as dried herb to be used for tea, and even pre-packaged into tea bags. These may not be pure ginseng products, though, since many teas contain sugar and other additives.

Tonics

Tonics are often of inferior quality, as are elixirs and mixed preparations with ginseng and other herbs or ingredients. These products often contain only minute amounts of ginseng.

Fresh and Dried Roots

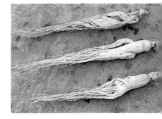

Fresh roots are usually treated with a lot of preservatives. Whole, dried roots are hard to chew. If they are saturated with honey, you can brake them into pieces at the dosage marks to make chewing easier. It is impossible to determine the purity of roots or the amount of active ingredients they contain.

When to Use Ginseng

Ginseng is a general tonic and a "cure-all" for almost anything. It is particularly well-suited for treating the chronic disorders of modern civilization in many industrialized countries.

Physical and Mental Stress

School exams, participation in competitive sports, stress at work or at home: these are only a few of the many life situations that can add up to too much strain on the organism. Toxins and radiation in the home or at work are environmental factors that can negatively effect energy levels and mental acuity. Harmful addictions, such as heavy smoking, exacerbate the problem.

People who are going through a stressful period in their lives or who suffer from lack of concentration, headaches, or fatigue can benefit from ginseng. This herb can increase the body's tolerance of

Main Applications at a Glance

Ailments:	Suggested Applications:
Chemotherapy, radiation	Ginseng cure before, during, and after
Chronic illness	Take ginseng daily on a long-term basis
Circulatory deficiencies	Take ginseng
Immune deficiency	Ginseng cure
Impotence	Ginseng cure
Physical or mental exhaustion	Ginseng cure
X-rays	Triple dose beforehand, and a four-week ginseng cure after exposure

stress and improve mental and physical stamina. Unlike synthetic sedatives, ginseng has a gentle, balancing effect that calms without making you feel as if you're in a fog, as artificial tranquilizers do. It also invigorates without over-stimulating.

Recipe

▶ Take ginseng before and during short periods of stress, such as an important deadline or meeting, an exam, a test, or a competitive sports event. Dosage: three grams daily for a week, then continue the cure for another four weeks at normal dose (one to two grams a day). Take a break (four weeks minimum), then repeat the cure if desired.

Chronic Illness

Ginseng reduces the side effects of chemo- or radiation therapy

Ginseng strengthens the immune system and reduces the incidence of colds. It also mobilizes the body's defenses against cancerous cells, making it useful in the prevention of various tumors.

Due to its regulatory function on the entire metabolism, ginseng can be used in conjunction with conventional medical treatments for a variety of diseases, including gout, rheumatoid conditions, high blood pressure, high cholesterol, arteriosclerosis, and diabetes. Patients usually report a significant reduction in secondary symptoms associated with these disorders, such as nervousness, insomnia, depression, fatigue, and general lack of energy. Used as a tonic after a serious illness, ginseng helps the body regain its strength and vitality.

Important: Ginseng can be used in conjunction with conventional medical treatments for all the diseases mentioned. However, discuss taking ginseng with your doctor first, and never discontinue your medication(s) or try to replace them with ginseng.

Important!

▶ *For prevention:*

If you are getting regular exercise and are eating a balanced diet, but feel that you want to do more to protect yourself from the diseases of modern civilization, you can periodically undergo a ginseng cure by taking one to two grams of ginseng a day for four weeks.

Recipes

▶ *Chronic illness:*

If you are suffering from a chronic illness, you can take one to two grams of ginseng a day on a regular basis, even for months or years. During periods of additional stress or aggravated health problems, you may want to temporarily increase the dosage to three to five grams a day for a week or two.

▶ *X-rays:*

Take a triple dose (three to six grams) of ginseng split into two doses on the two days before the procedure. After the x-rays, continue treatment with a normal dosage (one to two grams daily) for about four weeks, or, if chronically ill, longer.

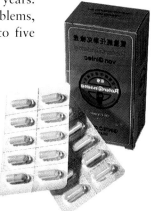

▶ *Chemo- or radiation therapy:*

For two days before starting therapy, take five grams of ginseng a day split into two doses. During therapy, take three grams a day. Following therapy, keep taking one to two grams of ginseng a day for at least a year.

Signs of Aging

Ginseng gently supports various regulatory functions in the body that tend to deteriorate with age. Women who take ginseng experience fewer or less severe symptoms when their bodies go through the hormonal changes of menopause. Ginseng root is also credited with mood enhancing properties, especially in the elderly.

▶ About twice a year, undergo a ginseng cure by taking one to two grams of ginseng a day for four weeks.

Recipe

Impotence

Impotence due to low sex drive, stress, or slightly reduced levels of sex hormones can be successfully treated with ginseng. The herb can increase male and female libido. In many cases, ginseng can even increase sperm count, and thus improve or restore fertility.

▶ Undergo a ginseng cure by taking two grams of ginseng every day for four weeks. Take a four-week break, then repeat the cure.

Recipe

Hawthorn

A Heart Tonic

Various species of hawthorn have been used in Chinese medicine for over a thousand years. In Europe, people were aware of the plant's medicinal properties during the Middle Ages, yet this knowledge was later forgotten. Superstition credited hawthorn with protective qualities: hung in doorways, its sprigs were said to drive off witches. Charms with hawthorn branches were believed to keep away illness.

Since the 19th century, herbal tea made from hawthorn flowers, leaves, and berries has again been used as a remedy for various heart ailments. The herb has also served as a treatment for coughs, kidney and urinary bladder ailments, and epilepsy. In recent years, hawthorn has finally achieved scientific recognition and has become one of the most popular herbs used in healing. It now plays an essential role as a heart remedy in naturopathic medicine.

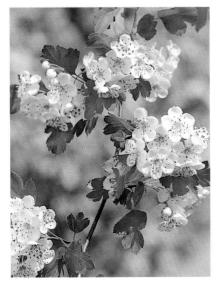

How to Identify Hawthorn

Hawthorn is a member of the rose family. Unfortunately, its flowers don't smell at all like roses, but more like herring brine! The two species of hawthorn used for medicinal purposes are single seed hawthorn (*Crataegus monogyna*), a shrub that grows up to twenty-five feet high and is often used for hedges, and English hawthorn (*Crataegus laevigata*), a tree that can reach a height of nearly forty feet. Both are native to Europe and North Africa, and are commonly grown as ornamental plants. In the wild, they prefer sunny slopes, thin underbrush, and deciduous forests as their habitat.

Hawthorn blossoms look strikingly beautiful but smell like herring brine

Hawthorn branches are covered with sharp thorns. The leaves, dark green on top and a paler greenish-blue on the underside, are three-lobed with irregularly serrated edges. From May to July, the plant carries white flowers with red stamens that later turn into red fruits. Hawthorn flowers and leaves taste slightly bitter, while its berries have a somewhat sweet flavor, are mealy, and contain quite a bit of mucilage.

How to Cultivate and Harvest Hawthorn

To grow a hawthorn hedge, plant cuttings measuring about six inches in two rows (place plants eighteen inches apart, with ten inches between rows). The soil should be rich in lime, but relatively poor in other nutrients.

Hawthorn should be picked fresh and used within a year. The tips of young shoots, about three inches in length, are harvested while the plant is in bloom. The berries are picked later on when they are bright red. All parts of the plant need to be dried quickly at temperatures not exceeding 113 degrees Fahrenheit. Once dried, the herb must be stored in tightly closed containers away from light and moisture. Improper storage may cause the loss of valuable active ingredients and reduce the herb's effectiveness as a remedy.

Due to its thorns, hawthorn used to be grown in hedges to serve as fencing around fields and pastures

What Makes Hawthorn So Valuable

Hawthorn is known for its gentle action. It is rich in flavonoids and contains various other active ingredients. Together, these chemical constituents improve circulation in the coronary blood vessels, strengthen the heart muscle, and regulate the discharge and transmission of electrical impulses in the heart. Due to these effects on the heart, hawthorn can also be helpful in correcting minor cardiac arrhythmia.

The herb has been shown to improve blood circulation in general. It also has a sedative effect and can relieve restlessness, insomnia, and the symptoms of menopause. Hawthorn helps prevent arteriosclerosis and helps to strengthen the body during recovery from illness.

Important: Never stop taking your prescription heart medication without consulting your doctor first. Sudden discontinuation of such drugs can lead to serious complications. Also, do not change the dosage of your medication unless instructed to do so by your physician.

Important!

How to Use Hawthorn

The dried herb available in health food or natural food stores consists either of flowers alone or of a mixture of flowers and leaves. Flowers alone are considerably more expensive and probably more effective than the mixture. On the other hand, research done on hawthorn has mainly focused on the mixed herb and its therapeutic effects.

Tea

You can use hawthorn flowers and leaves collected in the wild or in your garden, or purchase herb to prepare tea. Hawthorn tea is recommended as a remedy for minor heart ailments or as a means to prevent diminished heart function (myocardial insufficiency).

▶ *This is what you need:*
Hawthorn flowers and leaves, hot water

▶ *This is how it's done:*
Pour a cup of boiling water over a teaspoon of hawthorn flowers and leaves. Cover and let steep for twenty minutes, then strain.

Recipe

Additives for Flavoring
Hawthorn tea has very little flavor. You may want to sweeten it with honey or add a teaspoon of another herb, such as lemon balm, to give it a more interesting taste.

Drops

Recipe

A tincture can also be used as a general tonic to prevent diminished heart function, or as a remedy to relieve minor heart ailments. ▶ Fill a wide-necked bottle or large jar one-third full with fresh flowers and leaves. Add clear liquor to fill to the top. Keep in a warm, sunny place for six weeks, then strain.

Supplements

For more serious conditions, use hawthorn supplements available at health food stores. These products contain standardized amounts of the herb's active ingredients. The recommended dosage is 600 to 900 milligrams of powdered extract prepared from flowers and leaves.

Homeopathic Remedies

In homeopathy, "Crataegus" is mainly used as a basic tincture for heart ailments.

Hawthorn's red fruits are mealy and have a sweetish flavor

When to Use Hawthorn

Hawthorn develops its full therapeutic action slowly over the course of four to eight weeks. It is therefore necessary to take it for at least six weeks to see results.

✚ **See a doctor!**
Important: If you do not notice any improvement after six weeks of taking hawthorn, or if you develop edema in your legs, you must consult your doctor. If you experience shortness of breath or pain in the vicinity of the heart that radiates out into the arms, stomach area, or neck, see a doctor immediately.

Main Applications at a Glance

Ailments:	Suggested Applications:
Early stages of decreased heart function	Drink hawthorn tea or take extract
Neurocirculatory asthenia (weakness)	Drink tea made from herbal mixture

Prevention of Decreased Heart Function Due to Aging

After age thirty, human cardiovascular function steadily decreases. Reduced heart function, or myocardial insufficiency, is the most frequent diagnosis among patients over the age of sixty-five.

Hawthorn is excellent for prevention and treatment of slight myocardial insufficiency caused by weakness of the heart muscle due to aging, by an incipient decrease in circulation in the coronary blood vessels, or by acute infections, such as flu or pneumonia. As the heart gets stronger, related symptoms diminish, such as reduced stamina, shortness of breath, rapid fatigue, and coughing when stressed or tired. Hawthorn preparations are said to be so effective in treating mild myocardial insufficiency that they can compete with certain synthetic drugs, the so-called ACE-inhibitors.

► As you grow older, take 25 drops of hawthorn tincture one to three times a day, or drink a cup of hawthorn tea two to three times a day.

The best prevention is regular walking, swimming, or cycling

Recipe

Incipient Mild Myocardial Insufficiency

Early signs of reduced heart function are shortness of breath, rapid fatigue, quickened pulse, elevated blood pressure, and irregular heartbeat during normal activity. These symptoms disappear when the body is at rest.

► Drink three cups of hawthorn tea a day, or take 25 drops of tincture three times a day. If that's not convenient, or if you prefer a preparation with standardized amounts of active ingredients, take a commercially available extract according to instructions.

Recipe

Neurocirculatory Asthenia

These are heart problems that do not have an organic cause, but are brought on by stress or nervousness. The patient experiences chest pains, heart palpitations, quickened pulse, and increased sweating, along with nervousness and anxiety. Unlike heart ailments with organic causes, these symptoms are not brought on by physical exertion.

► Prepare a mixture of 20 grams of hawthorn (flowers and leaves), 10 grams of motherwort, 10 grams of lemon balm leaves, and 10 grams of valerian. Pour a cup of hot water over one to two teaspoons of herbal mixture. Let steep for ten minutes, then strain. Drink a cup of this tea, sweetened with honey, mornings and evenings until symptoms improve.

Recipe

Lavender

Relaxation for Body and Soul

Lavender's healing properties are first mentioned by Saint Hildegard in the 12th century. She refers to the herb as the "plant of the Virgin Mary," used as a remedy that "dispels impure thoughts and desires." Lavender also had other uses at the time, for instance as a treatment for dizziness, stroke, cramps, tremors, oral infections, and even edema. It was even said to act as a brain tonic when used in shampoos! In the meantime, the herb's beneficial effects on the brain and nervous system have been confirmed, though we no longer entertain the notion that they can be obtained by simply using a lavender shampoo. Today, we use lavender internally as a tea or inhale its volatile oils. The scent of lavender repels moths, so the herb is often used in linen closets.

How to Identify Genuine (English) Lavender

Lavender (*Lavandula angustifolia*) is a shrubby plant native to the warm, sunny slopes of the western Mediterranean region. It reaches a height of about 18 inches and has a woody rhizome. The rather long, thin leaves of the lavender plant are grayish-green in color and covered with silvery, felt-like hairs. Its purplish-blue flowers bloom between July and September and give off the characteristic lavender scent.

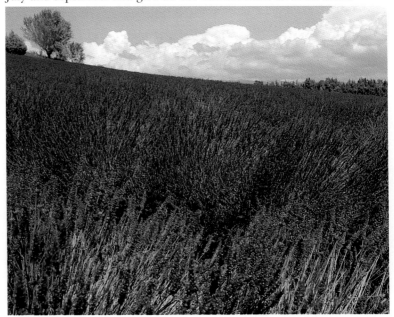

Lavender field in Provence (southern France)

How to Cultivate and Harvest Lavender

Lavender is a popular ornamental plant often used for landscaping. It is also grown commercially and processed into perfumes and oils. Large lavender fields are common in France, Spain, and eastern Europe. The evergreen shrub prefers very sunny locations and rich soil with plenty of lime. It is usually propagated through cuttings, but you can also plant seeds. Sow them in the spring and thin out the seedlings to allow about a foot between the individual plants. Lavender can also be grown in pots on a porch or balcony.

Planted next to vegetables, lavender acts as a natural pesticide

The herb is harvested when its flowers are in early bloom. Cut the stems with their flowering spikes, tie them into bundles, and hang them up to dry. The dried heads to be used for medicinal purposes are stripped from the stems and stored in tightly closed, dark glass jars to protect the herb from light and moisture.

What Makes Lavender So Effective

Lavender's main active ingredients are its volatile oils. The herb further contains tannins, bitters, and resins. Lavender calms frazzled nerves and is a fast-acting, dependable remedy for restlessness, nervousness, and insomnia. It is also useful as a treatment for nervous indigestion, abdominal gas, and loss of appetite, since these gastrointestinal problems are often caused by nervousness and stress. Lavender increases appetite by stimulating the production of bile. Baths with lavender are sometimes prescribed to treat circulatory problems or to promote healing of wounds.

An effective nerve tonic and a remedy for nervous indigestion

How to Use Lavender

Lavender can be drunk in the form of tea, or you can inhale its volatile oils. It can also be used in combination with other herbs that complement or enhance its medicinal effects.

Tea

▶ Pour a half-pint of boiling water over two teaspoons of lavender flowers. Let steep for five to ten minutes, then strain.

Recipes

Strong Tea

Strong tea is a popular additive for baths.
▶ Pour hot water over two to three ounces of lavender flowers.

Herbal Sachets

Mix equal parts of lavender flowers and hops and put the herbs into a linen sachet.

Essential Oils

These preparations contain volatile oils that have been extracted by steam distillation. Essential oils are either diffused with a vaporizer, taken internally, or added to massage oil.

Recipe ▶ Take one to four drops of lavender oil poured over a sugar cube.

When to Use Lavender

Lavender calms the nerves and is used to treat various ailments caused by stress and strain.

Main Applications at a Glance

Ailments:	Suggested Applications:
Circulatory problems, low blood pressure	Take a lavender bath
Digestive ailments	Drink lavender tea
Insomnia	Lavender bath, drink tea, herbal sachet
Intestinal problems due to nervousness	Drink lavender tea
Nervous exhaustion	Take a lavender bath, drink tea
Nervous indigestion	Drink lavender tea
Restlessness, nervousness	Take a lavender bath, drink tea

Nervous Exhaustion and Restlessness

At the end of an exhausting day, treat yourself to a relaxing evening: Turn off the television, unplug the phone, and take a fragrant, soothing lavender bath.

Recipe ▶ Add a strong tea prepared with lavender flowers to your bath water. Drink two cups of lavender tea sweetened with a teaspoon of honey. If you feel warm, you can also apply cold calf wraps (see page 160).

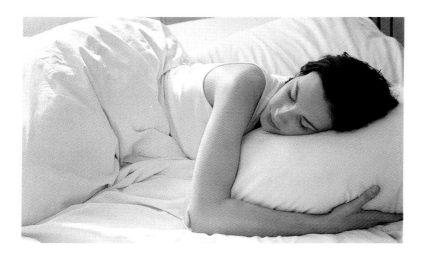

*Lavender calms
the nerves and
promotes restful
sleep*

Insomnia

Lavender taken at bedtime helps people fall asleep more quickly, and promotes longer and sounder sleep.

▶ Take a lavender bath in the evening, or drink one or two cups of lavender tea sweetened with honey an hour or two before bedtime. In addition, you can place an herbal sachet filled with lavender flowers and hops next to your pillow.

Recipe

Digestive Problems

Lavender flowers have a dual effect on the digestive system. They calm a nervous, irritable stomach and bowel and act as a digestive aid by stimulating the production of bile.

▶ For gastrointestinal complaints caused by nervousness or for other digestive ailments, drink three cups of lavender tea per day.

Recipe

Circulatory Problems

If you have low blood pressure or often feel dizzy due to circulatory problems, you should take advantage of the regulatory properties of lavender. Lavender baths are particularly helpful.

▶ For acute symptoms, take a lukewarm lavender bath. You can add a few drops of lavender oil to the bath water, or you can take the oil internally. Regular cold washings or affusions (see page 162) in the morning are also recommended.

Recipe

Mistletoe

An Ancient Remedy for Cancer

This herb is surrounded by many myths and legends. It is associated with the religious rites of the ancient Celtic Druids and was once thought to promote fertility and provide protection from poisons. The use of mistletoe as a medicinal plant goes back to the 5th century A.D.

Saint Hildegard of Bingen recommended European mistletoe grown on pear trees as a treatment for asthma, and in 16th century herbals it was mentioned as a remedy for epilepsy. Sebastian Kneipp administered European mistletoe to "stem blood flow and treat disorders of the circulatory system."

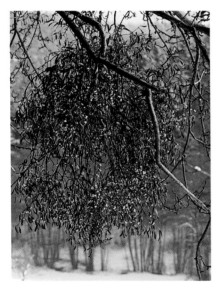

Mistletoe with berries growing on an apple tree

European mistletoe has long been used in folk medicine as a remedy for cancer. In 1916, Rudolf Steiner, the founder of the anthroposophical movement, developed a cancer therapy using mistletoe extracts. Conventional medicine still considers the use of this herb as a treatment for malignant tumors to be controversial.

How to Recognize European Mistletoe

European mistletoe (*Viscum album*) can be found throughout southern and central Europe as well as in parts of Asia. It should not be confused with American mistletoe, an entirely different plant species with some exactly opposite medicinal properties. European mistletoe is an evergreen semi-parasitic shrub that obtains most of the water and minerals needed for growth from its host tree. Branching freely, it forms into clumps or intricate balls of up to three feet in diameter. The plant can live to about seventy years. Mistletoe sprigs are olive green in color and have leathery leaves. Between March and April, inconspicuous, pale-yellow flowers appear in the forks of its twigs. The shrub's berry-like, pea-sized fruit doesn't ripen until December.

How to Cultivate and Harvest European Mistletoe

In Europe, an apple or pear tree grown in the garden can serve as a host for a mistletoe plant. Berries from a mistletoe sprig bought around Christmastime can be pressed into cracks in the bark of the tree. If the conditions are right, a seed will put down roots and grow into a plant.

Wild European mistletoe is usually found high up in treetops, and its form, a ball-shaped "nest," is very easy to make out when the tree is bare.

The parts of the plant used for medicinal purposes are the shoots including the leaves (but not the berries). They are picked either between March and April or between September and October, dried, and chopped.

Plant mistletoe on your apple tree

What Makes European Mistletoe So Valuable

According to research done in Germany, European mistletoe inhibits the growth of tumors and stimulates the immune system. These effects are said to be primarily due to chemical compounds called lectins. The herb also contains certain proteins (viscotoxins), flavonoids, resins, and mucilage. In combination, these active ingredients slightly reduce blood pressure, increase heart function, dilate blood vessels by relaxing their fine musculature, and have a calming effect on the nervous system. Injected into the skin, mistletoe preparations are believed to halt the progression of osteoarthritis, relieve the symptoms of whooping cough and asthma, and reduce dizziness.

European mistletoe preparations have also traditionally been used to treat women's ailments, such as scant menstrual flow and hot flashes, and as a means to prevent arteriosclerosis. The herb also serves as a heart tonic during recovery from serious illness.

A versatile herbal remedy

Undesirable Side Effects

Allergic reactions are possible, but they are rare. Injections into the skin may cause local irritation. The slight rise in body temperature generally caused by European mistletoe is considered to be desirable.

How to Use European Mistletoe

In addition to the preparations described in this chapter, there are numerous products that combine European mistletoe with other herbs. These mixtures are mainly used to lower elevated blood pressure or to treat various ailments typically associated with aging.

Injections

In Germany, mistletoe extracts obtained by various methods are sometimes injected intravenously to treat tumors. Extract is used as a therapy for osteoarthritis there as well. This requires injection under the skin. Neither treatment has been approved in the United States.

Tea

Recipe

▶ European mistletoe's stems and leaves require decoction to extract their active ingredients. Pour a cup of cold water over two teaspoons of finely chopped, dried herb. Let steep at room temperature for ten to twelve hours, then strain.

Tincture

Recipe

You can prepare your own European mistletoe tincture.
▶ Put fresh European mistletoe leaves into a dark glass jar with a screw-on lid. Add any distilled liquor or 70 percent (140 proof) alcohol to the top. Let the mixture steep for three weeks, shaking it well once a day. Press out the leaves. Filter the liquid through a thin cloth and pour it into small bottles. Take twenty drops of the tincture three times a day. This is equivalent to two cups of tea.

Supplements and Homeopathic Remedies

These preparations are available from some natural food stores and suppliers of herbs.

A homeopathic remedy for the elderly

The homeopathic remedy "Viscum album" contains mistletoe and is often prescribed for elderly patients as a tonic or a treatment for poor blood circulation in the arms and legs.

When to Use European Mistletoe

European mistletoe is an effective remedy for preventing and treating chronic ailments of the cardiovascular system and the joints. As an alternative to mistletoe tea or tincture as described in recipes, you can also take supplements (for proper dosage, follow the instructions on the product's label).

The Main Applications at a Glance

Ailments:	Suggested Applications:
Arteriosclerosis	A cure with European mistletoe tea
Cardiovascular problems	A cure with European mistletoe tea
Malignant tumors	Treatment with injections (Not available in the United States)
Osteoarthritis	A cure with European mistletoe tea; injections (Not available in the U.S.)

Tumors

Studies conducted in Germany have shown that European mistletoe extract can inhibit the growth of tumors. As an added benefit, treatment with mistletoe often significantly improves the patient's general sense of well-being as well. This may be due to the herb's anxiety reducing properties. It needs to be pointed out that while therapies employing extract—administered only by a physician— appear to be promising, drinking mistletoe tea is not an effective treatment for tumors!

A cure with European mistletoe tea helps with arteriosclerosis

Osteoarthritis

"Segment therapy" is a form of therapeutic anesthesia where mistletoe extract is injected into the skin by experienced practitioners. It often halts the progressive joint degeneration associated with osteoarthritis. Undergoing regular cures with European mistletoe tea in conjunction with injections is recommended.

▶ Prepare a tea using two pints of cold water and four teaspoons of dried European mistletoe leaves. It is best to brew the tea in the evening, let it steep overnight, and drink one cup in the morning and one at night. Do this daily for about four weeks.

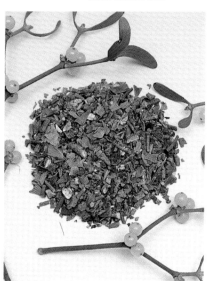

Cardiovascular Disease

Trying some European mistletoe tea or tincture is worthwhile for people suffering from slightly elevated blood pressure (borderline hypertension) or mild neurocirculatory asthenia. European mistletoe is also used for the prevention and treatment of arteriosclerosis.

▶ *Slightly elevated blood pressure:*
Drink one to two cups of mistletoe tea a day for about two months. Have your blood pressure checked regularly at your doctor's office.

▶ *Mild neurocirculatory asthenia:*
After you have seen a doctor, drink two to three cups of European mistletoe tea for about two weeks. If symptoms persist or worsen, seek medical attention immediately.

▶ *Arteriosclerosis:*
Drink one to two cups of European mistletoe tea daily for four weeks. Repeat this cure at least twice a year.

Recipes

✚ **See a doctor**

St. John's Wort

A Natural Mood Enhancer

Centuries ago, St. John's wort was known as the *sun plant*, an herb capable of warding off demons and lifting dark moods. The plant is said to have come from the blood of Saint John the Baptist. Numerous myths and legends have sprung up around the herb, crediting it with the power to avert black magic, exorcise the devil, and undo the spells of witches.

Paracelsus sang the praises of St. John's wort more than 450 years ago, extolling its "...healing effects on wounds, broken bones, and all manners of despondency..." At that time, the plant was one of the most popular and well-known herbal remedies, used for dressing wounds and ulcers, and serving as a treatment for depression, lumbago, and menstrual problems. In recent years, clinical tests have confirmed some of St. John's wort's medicinal properties, especially its effect as a mood enhancer. These results have received much attention and have once more made St. John's wort one of the most popular remedies available.

How to Recognize Common St. John's Wort

St. John's wort (*Hypericum perforatum*) can be found throughout much of Europe and western Asia. It prefers dry, chalky or loamy soil,

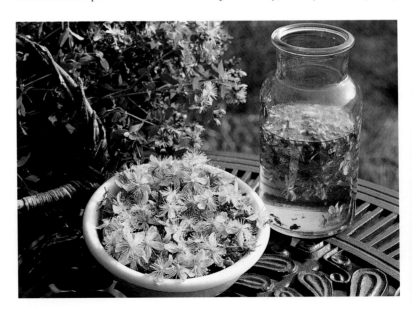

St. John's wort flowers, dried and suspended in oil

and thrives on railroad embankments, riverbanks, roadsides, and on the edges of forests. The herb grows to a height of about three feet. Only Common St. John's wort is used for medicinal purposes. You can recognize it by its unique stems and leaves: the stems have two raised ridges, and the leaves, when held up to the light, appear to be punctured by small holes. (The "holes" are actually translucent oil glands.)

The peak of the plant's flowering season falls into the period around the birthday of Saint John the Baptist on June 24th. The flower's bright yellow petals have small black dots and yield a bluish-red dye when crushed.

Another common name is gout weed

Cultivating and Harvesting St. John's Wort

This plant, with its golden yellow flowers, will thrive in your garden. You can start it from seeds that you plant in shallow containers around the end of March. Keep the containers in a warm, sunny spot, and make sure that the soil is always slightly moist. When the seedlings are almost two inches tall, transplant the healthiest ones to a sunny area in your garden. Space them about a foot apart. You can also buy St. John's wort plants from a nursery.

The herb is best harvested within a few days before or after St. John's day, since this is the time when it is said to be richest in chemically active ingredients, and therefore most potent as a remedy. Choose tender tops with flowers and cut them close to the ground with a knife or with pruning shears. Tie the herbs into loose bunches and hang them up to dry in an airy, shaded place.

What Makes St. John's Wort So Valuable

Saint John's wort's main active ingredient is hypericin. This chemical compound is found in the red dye secreted by its flower petals when they are crushed. Other constituents present in all the tops of the plant are hyperforin, which together with hypericin is believed to be responsible for the herb's antidepressant effect, and other compounds, such as flavonoids, tannins, and volatile oils.

The herb's most remarkable characteristic is its action on the nervous system and the brain. It seems to inhibit the body's reaction to strong neuronal stimuli and to lift depressed moods. Clinical trials have shown that St. John's wort is as effective in treating mild to moderate depression as the synthetic drugs (antidepressants) commonly used. Yet unlike these drugs, St. John's wort hardly causes any undesirable side effects.

There is no risk of dependency

St. John's wort also has other medicinal uses. It promotes healing of wounds, relieves pain, stimulates the secretion of gastric juices, and is said to inhibit the reproduction of viruses.

Undesirable Side Effects

One possible side effect of St. John's wort is increased photosensitivity. When taking the herb, very fair-skinned people should avoid sunbathing in bright sun and stay away from tanning salons. Skin covered with St. John's wort oil should not be exposed to the sun.

How to Use St. John's Wort

St. John's wort is equally effective whether taken as a tea or tincture or applied as an oil. Standardized, commercially produced preparations provide the highest, most consistent concentrations of chemically active ingredients.

Tea

You can prepare St. John's wort tea from your own flowers and leaves or buy dried herb. The tea can be steeped in either hot or cold water. Infusions—preparations with hot water—taste better than decoctions—where cold water is poured over the herb—because they contain fewer tannins. Infusions are also generally easier for the body to tolerate.

Recipes

▶ **Infusion:** Pour a cup of boiling water over one to two teaspoons of finely chopped, dried herb. Cover to prevent the volatile oils from escaping. Let steep for ten minutes, then strain. Sweeten with honey if desired. Drink warm.

▶ **Decoction:** Measure one to two teaspoons of finely chopped, dried herb into a ceramic pot and add a large cup of cold water. Cover and bring to a boil. Reduce the heat and let simmer for five minutes, then strain. Drink warm.

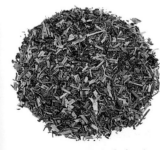

Infused Red Oil

St. John's wort oil is made from fresh flowers. You can prepare your own oil or buy it at a health food store.

▶ *This is what you need:*
Fresh St. John's wort buds or flowers, olive oil

▶ *This is how it's done:*
Crush two handfuls of freshly opened flowers with a mortar and pestle and put them into a large screw-top jar or bottle of clear glass. The herb should take up about a third of the space in the jar. Fill to the top with olive oil. Keep the tightly closed jar in a warm, sunny spot for about four weeks.

*Dried, finely
chopped St.
John's wort for
making tea*

The oil will turn bright red. Strain it through a thin cloth, then pour it into small glass bottles and store them in a dark place.

Tip

Apply to Warm Skin
When using St. John's wort oil externally, massage the affected area first to warm it up before applying the oil. This will improve its absorption into the skin.

Tincture

Here's another preparation you can either make yourself or buy at a health food store.

► *This is what you need:*
Fresh or dried herb, half a quart of 70% percent (140-proof) alcohol

► *This is how it's done:*
Pour the alcohol over a handful of fresh or dried herb. Let steep in a tightly closed jar or bottle for two weeks. Keep the jar or bottle in a dark place and shake it well from time to time. Strain through a thin cloth and press all the liquid out of the herb. Store the finished tincture in a tightly closed, dark glass bottle in a dark place.

Recipe

Supplements

Standardized, highly concentrated extract used for treating depression is sold in health food and natural food stores. Processed into powder and usually sold in capsule form, this extract contains a certified amount of active ingredients. Take one gram of powdered St. John's wort extract per day.

Facial Steam Bath

► Put a handful of dried St. John's wort into a bowl. Pour about two quarts of hot water over the herb. Lean over the bowl and drape a towel over your head and the bowl. Inhale the rising vapors for about ten minutes.

Recipe

Important: Due to the danger of scalding, never leave children unattended while they inhale!

Important!

Homeopathic Remedies

St. John's wort is also used in homeopathy for treating wounds, injured nerves, neuralgia, and depression.

When to Use St. John's Wort

St. John's wort has many medicinal uses. It primarily serves as a treatment for depression and ailments characterized by anxiety or nervousness.

Main Applications at a Glance

Ailments:	Suggested Applications:
Abdominal gas in children	Drink tea
Back pain	Warm compresses with oil
Bed wetting in children	Tea; massage oil into stomach and inner thighs
Cold sores	Dab with oil
Depression	Drink tea or take a supplement
Insomnia	Take tea or a supplement; warm stomach wraps
Lack of concentration, nervousness	Drink tea or take a supplement
Muscle pain	Massage and apply warm oil compresses
Neuralgia	Take tea or a supplement; warm compresses
Shingles	Dab with oil, take tea or a supplement
Sunburn, mild burns	Apply oil
Wounds	Compresses, apply oil

Psychological Disorders

Depression, persistent fatigue, lack of motivation, and poor concentration are all common symptoms of depression. Often accompanied by insomnia and changes in appetite, they frequently occur during the winter months when our bodies are exposed to less natural light (seasonal affective disorder or SAD). Going for walks in fresh air and taking St. John's wort can lift minor depression in most cases. The herb's calming properties also help relieve mild anxiety and the mental stress prior to exams that can sometimes lead to insomnia.

Treatment with St. John's wort requires patience. Although some improvement may be felt immediately, it usually takes three weeks for the herb to take effect.

✚ See a doctor

Recipes

▶ *Slightly depressed mood:*
Prepare an infusion or decoction with Saint John's wort as described above. Drink two to three cups of the tea per day, especially during the winter months. If you have suffered from seasonal affective disorder in the past, it's a good idea to start this tea cure as a preventive measure in October.

▶ *Mild to moderate depression:*
If depressive symptoms as described above affect your everyday life, use concentrated St. John's wort extract in powder or capsule form, available at your health food or natural food store.

▶ *Insomnia:*
Buy herbs in bulk from a natural food store and prepare the following customized tea mixture: 20 grams of St. John's wort, 10 grams of lemon balm, 10 grams of hops, and 10 grams of lavender. Pour a cup of hot water over a heaping teaspoon of the herb mixture and drink this tea one hour before bedtime.

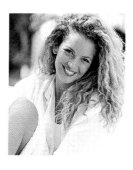

An even temperament and optimism through St. John's wort

Wounds and Burns

In folk medicine, St. John's wort has enjoyed an excellent, long-standing reputation as a remedy for rashes, skin ulcers, acne, sharp or blunt puncture wounds, and sunburn. The oil in particular promotes healing and has anti-bacterial and analgesic properties.

▶ *Wounds:*
Saturate several layers of gauze bandage with red oil and apply them to the wound. Repeat the treatment every two hours.

▶ *Sunburn:*
Allow mild burns to cool off first. For that purpose, wet a hand towel, wring it out, and apply it to the affected area. As an alternative, you can apply a half-inch layer of firm plain yogurt (drain it if necessary). When the skin feels reasonably cool, remove the hand towel or yogurt. Carefully apply St. John's wort oil to the reddened area. Repeat three times a day or as needed.

Recipes

Muscle Pain and Neuralgia

St. John's wort oil relieves muscle pain due to conditions such as a tight or pulled muscle or a rheumatoid disorder. Various kinds of neuralgia, such as trigeminal nerve pain, sciatic pain, and lumbago, also respond well to treatment with St. John's wort.

Recipe

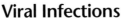

▶ *Bruises and pulled muscles:*
Gently apply St. John's wort oil to the affected areas several times a day, and if they're not too tender, carefully massage it in.

Viral Infections

In addition to its action as an analgesic and a muscle relaxant, St. John's wort also appears to have antiviral properties. For this reason, it has long been used in folk medicine as a treatment for herpes infections.

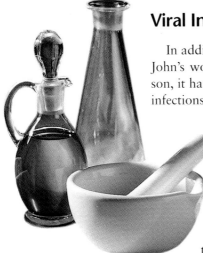

▶ *Shingles:*
Use St. John's wort in conjunction with conventional medical treatment. Carefully apply St. John's wort oil to the affected area. It's a good idea to wear an old undershirt to protect your outer clothing from oil stains.

▶ *Cold sores:*
At the first sign of blisters, apply St. John's wort oil or tincture. Keep the affected area moist. This usually keeps the condition from becoming painful.

Pediatric Uses

St. John's wort is very effective in relieving stomachaches and bed wetting. It is very well tolerated and entirely safe for children.

Recipes

▶ *Abdominal gas or nonspecific stomachaches:*
Massage St. John's wort oil into the baby's or toddler's stomach area, using clockwise, circular strokes. This treatment can be preceded by a warm bath.

▶ *Bed wetting:*
This condition is often a symptom of an emotional problem. Have the child drink a cup of St. John's wort tea in the early afternoon. Sweeten the tea with honey if desired. In addition, massage St. John's wort oil into the child's lower abdomen and inner thighs at bedtime. This helps prevent chafing of the skin and heightens the sensitivity of the pelvic muscles, which play a role in bladder control.

Stinging Nettle

For Health and Beauty

The stinging nettle is often cursed as an annoying weed by people who are unaware of its remarkable healing properties. It has primarily served as a diuretic and as a remedy for ailing joints. More recently, the roots of the stinging nettle plant are used to alleviate symptoms associated with benign enlargement of the prostate gland.

Large stinging nettles with flowers

How to Identify Stinging Nettle

Nettle leaves have coarsely serrated edges that are covered on both sides with stinging hairs. When we brush against them, these hairs break off, become lodged in our skin, and produce the familiar, uncomfortable burning sensation. This property distinguishes the large and small stinging nettle from the white dead nettle, which does not cause burning, itchy skin. Large stinging nettle (*Urtica dioica*), a perennial, reaches a height of up to almost six feet and produces small greenish flowers. Small stinging nettle (*Urtica urens*) only grows to about three feet tall. Both species produce small, nut-like fruits. When ripe, the fruits are sandy brown in color and smell like carrots.

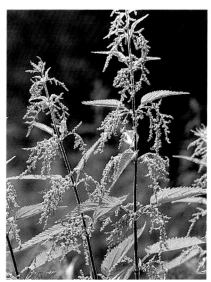

How to Cultivate and Harvest Stinging Nettle

Small stinging nettle causes more severe burning than large nettle

Stinging nettle can be grown from seeds that are planted in May or June. Sowing them earlier is not recommended since they require high soil temperatures in order to sprout. For best results, cover the ground with thin, light-colored netting after you have planted the seeds. Stinging nettle can also be propagated by dividing the root in two and planting each half as a separate plant.

Young shoots are harvested for preparing fresh juice, and the entire tops are used to produce dried herb. When nettle plants are at least three years old, their roots are mature enough to be collected. This should be done in the fall or spring. The fruits are picked from September to October.

Dried fruits are best stored in a cardboard box

What Makes Stinging Nettle So Effective

The tops of stinging nettle are very rich in tannins, minerals (especially iron), vitamins A and C, and flavonoids. The fruits contain proteins, mucilage, and high amounts of unsaturated fatty acids. The stinging hairs produce their notorious burning effect by injecting small amounts of acetylcholine, serotonin, and formic acid into the skin. Stinging nettle acts primarily as a diuretic. It also stimulates the production of red blood cells and bile, and is an effective expectorant. Due to its tannins, the herb has traditionally been used as a treatment for stomach ailments and diarrhea. Beta-sitosterol, found in the roots, is the active ingredient responsible for the plant's ability to relieve various symptoms associated with benign enlargement of the prostate. Stinging nettle fruits are particularly recommended as a tonic for older patients.

Undesirable Side Effects

✚ See a doctor

Used internally, stinging nettle roots can occasionally cause mild gastrointestinal complaints. Never use stinging nettle to treat edema due to impaired heart or kidney function. Always consult a doctor if you suffer from heart or kidney disease.

How to Use Stinging Nettle

Since stinging nettle grows almost everywhere, in the spring and summer you can make many of the following remedies yourself. Various nettle preparations and supplements are also available in health food and natural food stores.

Tea

Recipes

▶ **Infusion:** Pour a cup of hot water over one to two teaspoons of dried herb. Let steep for ten minutes, then strain.
▶ **Decoction:** Measure one to two teaspoons of chopped, dried stinging nettle root into a ceramic pot. Add a large cup of cold water. Cover and bring to a boil. After about a minute, remove the pot from the burner. Keep the tea covered and let it steep for ten minutes, then strain.

Tincture

Recipe

▶ Wash fresh roots, mince them, and put them into a glass jar with a screw-on lid. Add 45 percent alcohol until the roots are covered.

Close the jar tightly and let steep for three weeks, shaking the mixture from time to time. Strain and pour into dark glass bottles.

Stinging nettle tincture is also commercially available.

Stinging Nettle Juice

Stinging nettle juice should be prepared fresh in a juicer every day. This is the most effective form of the herb.

▶ Always dilute stinging nettle juice. Use one part juice to five parts of water. Instead of water, you can also use buttermilk.

Keeping a Ready Supply of Leaves
If you can't gather fresh stinging nettle leaves on a daily basis, keep a supply handy that lasts you for a while. Wrapped in moist kitchen towels and stored in the refrigerator, nettle leaves will stay fresh for a few days.

Fruits

▶ Stinging nettle fruits ground in a pepper or coffee mill or crushed with a mortar and pestle can be used internally or applied as a poultice (see page 161).

Supplements

Beta-sitosterol, the active ingredient used to treat benign enlargement of the prostate, is contained in the roots of the stinging nettle plant. Nettle root extract is commercially produced, and can be purchased in capsule form from health food and natural food stores.

Spirits

Stinging nettle spirit, which is massaged into affected joints to relieve gout and rheumatic complaints, is available in health food stores.

Homeopathic Preparations

The homeopathic remedy Urtica urens is prepared from small stinging nettle. It is used to treat allergic skin conditions related to urticaria, commonly known as hives or nettle rash, as well as for kidney ailments and gout.

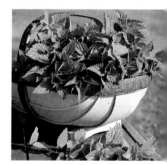

Freshly picked stinging nettle leaves can be eaten as a salad

When to Use Stinging Nettle

Preparations made from stinging nettle are mainly used for treating kidney, bladder, and prostate ailments. They also serve as a tonic for patients suffering from general exhaustion.

Main Applications at a Glance

Ailments:	Suggested Applications:
Blemished skin	Take a cure of stinging nettle tea
Enlargement of the prostate	Take a supplement or tincture
Gout	Drink tea, eat fruits or apply them as a poultice; massage spirit of stinging nettle into joints
Hair loss, dandruff	Rinse hair with stinging nettle decoction
Rheumatoid conditions	Drink tea, eat fruits or apply them as a poultice, massage spirit of stinging nettle into joints
Small kidney stones	Drink stinging nettle tea
Spring fatigue	Take a cure with fresh nettle juice
Urinary bladder infection	Drink stinging nettle tea

Seasonal Fatigue, Exhaustion

A cure with fresh stinging nettle juice or ground nettle fruits acts as a general tonic, and is recommended for seasonal fatigue or exhaustion due to mental or emotional stress or a long term illness.

Recipe

▶ Start by taking three tablespoons of stinging nettle juice per day. After three days, increase the dosage by one tablespoon. Continue adding another tablespoon every three days to a maximum dosage of ten tablespoons per day.

T!p

Mix and Match!
For a fresh juice cure, combine stinging nettle with other herbs, such as dandelion, ribwort, horsetail or bottlebrush, watercress, Saint John's wort, hops, alpine wild garlic (also called bear paw garlic), angelica, or even a few feverfew flowers. Half of the juice should be stinging nettle, the other half can consist of herbs of your choice.

Urinary Tract Disorders

Stinging nettle tea is ideally suited for flushing out the urinary tract when suffering from an urinary bladder infection, or for preventing or treating small kidney stones. For all urinary tract disorders, it's essential to drink lots of fluids.
▶ Drink at least six to eight cups of stinging nettle tea a day.

Recipe

Enlargement of the Prostate (prostate hypertrophy)

The symptoms of benign enlargement of the prostate consist of difficulties in emptying the bladder, such as impaired urinary flow or a frequent urge to urinate.

The disease must be diagnosed by a physician. If it is in its early stages, herbal remedies are usually effective in relieving the symptoms.
▶ Take either a commercially available stinging nettle preparation on a daily basis according to the directions on the label, or 20 drops of stinging nettle tincture three times a day.

This condition requires regular checkups by a physician

Recipe

Rheumatoid Conditions and Gout

If you suffer from gout or from a rheumatoid disorder that affects your joints and muscles, you should, along with using stinging nettle preparations externally, take steps to flush uric acid out of your body.
▶ Take a three-week cure with stinging nettle by either drinking five cups of tea or eating one to two tablespoons of crushed nettle fruits daily. Massage the painful joints and muscles with stinging nettle spirit, or apply a poultice of crushed nettle fruits.

Recipe

Skin and Hair

Stinging nettle detoxifies and purifies the blood. These properties make it particularly suitable for treating blemished skin. Stinging nettle can also be used in the form of Kneipp's hair tonic.
▶ *Blemished skin:*
Take a stinging nettle cure by drinking four to six cups of tea, or take fresh nettle juice (as recommended for seasonal fatigue) daily for four weeks.
▶ *Hair loss, dandruff:*
To prepare Kneipp's hair tonic, boil seven ounces of freshly picked stinging nettle leaves for a half-hour in a quart of water, then strain. Massage the tonic into your hair and scalp at bedtime.

Caution: Stinging nettle stock can discolor light hair

Recipes

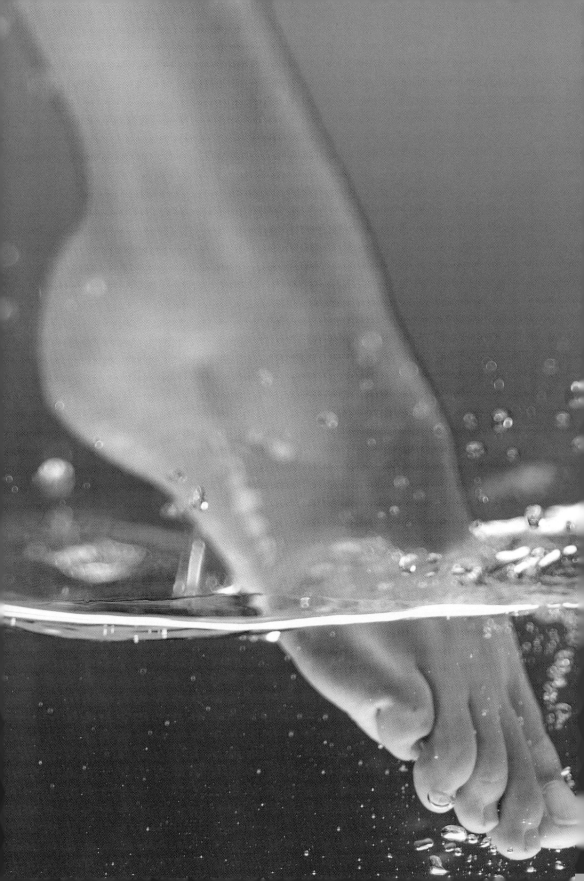

Hydrotherapy

Water is essential for our existence. Without it, there would be no life. We feel comfortable in water from birth. It is gentle and pure as it emerges from the earth as a mountain spring, awe-inspiring as it crashes down a waterfall, or boiling hot as it spews forth from a geyser. It can be translucent and plain, taste of salt, iron, or chalk, reek of sulfur, or be naturally sparkling.

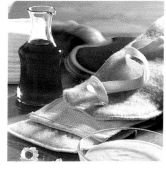

Water can be used in all its varied forms to promote health. The knowledge of its healing powers represents one of the earliest medical discoveries. Water that is naturally rich in minerals is not only wholesome when taken internally, but when used externally for various applications, it also has healing properties that can benefit the entire body. What's more, water produces no undesirable side effects. In the following chapter you will learn how to use water to prevent, relieve, or cure various ailments. You are invited to discover a type of medical treatment that can actually be fun.

The Healing Powers of Water

People first discovered the healing powers of water around the time of Hippocrates, several centuries before the birth of Christ. The ancient Chinese and Romans promoted bathing and were quite advanced in their knowledge of its uses and potential benefits. In the Middle Ages, the culture of bathing was abandoned in an effort to stem the spread of venereal disease, the "scourge of lust." The healing powers of water were rediscovered in the 19th century by Sebastian Kneipp, a German priest and healer. Suffering from tuberculosis, a disease considered incurable at the time, he treated himself with various water applications and eventually recovered from his illness. As a result, he devoted thirty years of his life to research

Water is one of the most powerful forces in nature; without water, there is no life

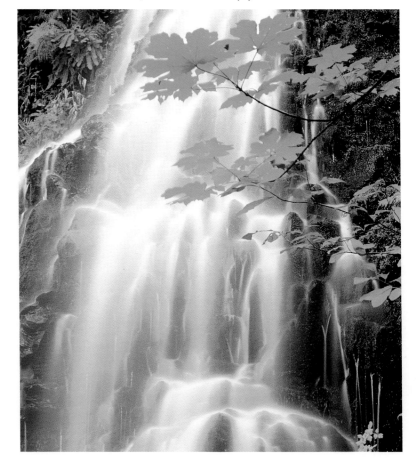

and to refining the methods of what is known today as Kneipp's water cure or hydrotherapy. It took a while for medical doctors to accept his ideas. Today, Kneipp's hydrotherapy is still used pretty much in its original form. What has changed is that we now have running hot water, a modern convenience that makes water applications considerably easier.

How to Use Hydrotherapy

Although hydrotherapy is an external treatment, it affects the entire body. As a first reaction to cold water, the blood vessels in and beneath the skin contract to prevent the loss of heat. Once the cold stimulus diminishes, the blood vessels dilate considerably to allow sufficient amounts of oxygen and nutrients to reach the temporarily starved surface of the body. This leads to increased respiratory and metabolic function, strengthens the lymphatic and immune systems, and through the nerves, stimulates the internal organs.

In addition, water affects the functioning of the autonomic nervous system, the production of hormones, and body temperature. It also improves the elasticity of the skin.

The body learns to react faster to changes in temperature

Hydrotherapy is used to treat a variety of disorders. Stimuli provided by cold water are more effective for acute conditions. They raise the pain threshold, stem acute infections, and increase respiration. Warm water is more useful in treating chronic ailments. It is recommended for patients who feel very weak or cold. Heat relaxes the bronchi and gently supports the body in fighting illness.

How to Use Water

Water can be used in its solid, liquid, or gaseous state and is readily available to anyone. The treatment can be adjusted to the condition and the needs of each patient. If a person is weak due to surgery or serious illness, the difference in temperature and the force of the water are decreased to provide a milder stimulus.

The intensity of the stimulus provided by the water is dependent upon its temperature, the duration of the treatment, and the size of the area of the body to which the water is applied. People who are not used to cold should start with mild stimulation when using cold water applications. The body needs time to adjust to lower temperatures. One way to accomplish this is by starting with affusions to the knees, then proceeding to the thighs, then to the body below the waist, and finally to the whole body. For cold packs, the water temperature should initially be between 72 and 75 degrees Fahrenheit.

Cold water provides stronger stimuli than warm water

After several applications, the temperature can be gradually lowered. The reverse is true for baths. Here, water temperatures for subsequent applications should get increasingly warmer.

As a rule, hydrotherapy should never be uncomfortable. Cold parts of the body must be warmed up gradually and gently, even in people who are used to cold. When the body is warm or overheated, both warm and cold applications are appropriate.

Children are more sensitive and react much more strongly than adults to the stimuli provided by hydrotherapy. When treating ailments that would normally call for cold applications, use lukewarm instead of cold water for small children. In general, the water temperature should be only a few degrees cooler than the child's body temperature.

Follow these Guidelines
- Hydrotherapy should be done in a room that is well ventilated and warm.
- Do not do hydrotherapy shortly before or after a meal.
- Keep breathing regularly during the treatment. Do not hold your breath.
- After the treatment, don't dry your body off with a towel. Wipe the water off with your hands instead, then lay down in your bed and get warm. After a knee affusion, mild exercise is a good way to get warm.

✚ See a doctor

Important: If you are nauseous, have a severe headache, are exhausted, or experience chest pain, use only very gentle applications. If symptoms don't improve within a day, or if they get worse, you should see your doctor. Bedridden or chronically ill people should undergo hydrother-apy only with the approval of a qualified health care professional.

Undesirable Side Effects

In general, hydrotherapy produces no undesirable side effects. However, people who suffer from cardiovascular ailments or poor blood circulation should avoid applications that provide strong temperature stimuli, such as hot baths or full body affusions. Do not apply local heat to tumors. If bath salts or other ingredients are added to the water used, allergic reactions to these substances are possible. In that case, discontinue the therapy.

Wraps

Wraps are versatile and very easy to apply. However, they require time: A wrap should be left on for half an hour to an hour, and the patient should spend the same amount of time resting after the wrap has been removed.

Wraps are usually applied to the part of the body that is ailing. They are differentiated according to temperature and to their desired effect. Most wraps are cold. Cold temperatures initially cause the blood vessels to contract, then to dilate. The skin gets warm. The effects of cold wraps can be intensified by adding various ingredients to the water.

With a little practice, wraps are easy to apply

> **Different Kinds of Applications**
> ● Packs are simply placed on the affected area
> ● Compresses are small packs
> ● Large packs cover over half of the body

Important: Warm wraps should not be used on patients with a fever. Cold wraps are not recommended if the patient feels cold or if the body part to be treated is cold.

Preparation

Provide an environment that promotes relaxation. Allow enough time for the treatment and for a resting period afterwards. Before you start, use the bathroom if needed. The room should be well ventilated and comfortably warm. The patient should always lie down for a wrap. Arrange everything you will need within easy reach so that the wrap can be applied quickly.

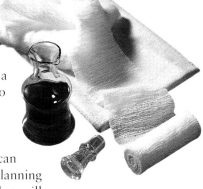

▶ *This is what you need:*
● An inner cloth or towel made of linen or cotton. (You can use old sheets, dish towels, or cloth diapers.) If you are planning to apply a poultice (such as ground mustard or onion) that will not come in direct contact with the skin, this inner towel should be three times the size of the affected area.
● An intermediate cotton towel that is large enough to cover the wet inner layer completely. Instead of a separate intermediate towel, you can use a double sized towel that serves both as an inner and an intermediate layer. In this case, soak one-half of the inner towel in the liquid you are using and leave the other half dry. Place the wet part onto the skin and fold the dry part over it.

- An outer layer of wool fabric that is large enough to wrap around the body part being treated.
- Ingredients to be used for a poultice (if desired), such as drained plain yogurt, clay, mashed potato, ground mustard seed, or onions.
- First-aid tape, bandage clips, or bandages for holding the wrap in place.
- A blanket to keep the patient warm.

Special Wool for Added Warmth
Instead of an intermediate towel you can use pure, raw sheep's wool for added warmth. This wool comes in layers and is sometimes sold in drug stores or in stores that sell wool yarns.

▶ *This is how it's done:*
- Dip the inner towel in the liquid you are using for the wrap. Wring it out so it no longer drips. If you're using a poultice that's not supposed to be applied directly to the skin, use a towel that's three times the size of the area you want to cover with the poultice. Spread the paste, such as mashed potato, ground mustard, or onion, onto the middle third of the towel, leaving equal space to the left and right. Fold over the outer two-thirds of the towel and place the pack face down onto the affected area. The single layer of fabric between the body and the poultice will allow enough of the active ingredients in the paste to penetrate to the skin. Apply the wrap in a manner that insures full contact with the body without any gaps or folds.
- Cover the inner towel with the intermediate towel. It should be pulled tight but not be too restricting. Now wrap the wool towel around the body part you are treating. Wool that comes in direct contact with the skin sometimes causes irritation. You can avoid this by using an intermediate towel that's large enough to fold back over the edges of the woolen towel.
- Fasten the wrap with first-aid tape, bandage clips, or gauze bandages.
- Cover the patient well to preserve warmth.

Cold Wraps and Wraps at Body Temperature

Cold wraps improve blood circulation, increase blood flow to the area of the body being treated, promote the excretion of metabolic waste products through the skin, and have a generally calming effect. Except in the case of a fever, they are intended to generate warmth. After about ten minutes, a cold wrap usually begins to feel warm. If this isn't the case, a hot water bottle or hot tea can be used to warm up the patient.

The water temperature should be from about 62 to 72 degrees Fahrenheit

T¡p

Poultices Need Not Be Applied Directly to the Skin
When applying a poultice, first place a layer of bandage
or gauze from the drugstore onto the skin, then add the
paste, such as mineral-rich clay. Finally, add the wrap itself.
This method will make it easier to remove the paste later.

Wraps are left on the body for about half an hour to an hour,
until the area being treated is thoroughly warm. Wraps that are primarily used to calm the patient can be left on overnight. Those that
are intended to cool, like wraps applied to insect bites, bruises, or
inflamed joints, or those given to a patient with a fever, should be
changed every ten minutes.

Ingredients Used for Cold Wraps

Recipes

Apple cider vinegar
- increases the stimulating effect on the vascular system, relieves
  itching, has a cooling effect
- for insect bites and tired, aching legs

▶ *This is how it's done:*
Prepare a mixture of 20 tablespoons of pure apple cider vinegar and
a quart of cold water. The inner towel used for the wrap is soaked
in this liquid.

Mineral-rich clay
- relieves inflammation
- soothes irritated, inflamed skin and rashes

▶ *This is how it's done:*
Mix three tablespoons of clay with water to make a firm paste.
Chill, then apply a quarter-inch layer to the inner towel and place
it face down onto the skin.

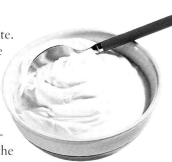

Salt
- increases the stimulating effect of the wrap; extracts water
  from the body
- relieves swelling and reduces edema in the tissues; recommended for venous insufficiency to restore tone and elasticity to the
  walls of the veins

▶ *This is how it's done:*
Stir four teaspoons of sea salt into a quart of cold water. Use this
liquid for your wrap.

Yogurt
Use well-drained, firm plain yogurt.
- has a cooling, soothing effect, moisturizes the skin and relieves pain
- relieves acute inflammation, reduces swelling; helpful for sunburns

▶ *This is how it's done:*
Spread a quarter-inch thick layer of yogurt onto the inner towel used for the wrap and place it face down onto the skin.

Warm Wraps

When the body's regenerative powers can no longer be mobilized by cold wraps, it is necessary to turn to warm wraps. This type of application is always appropriate when the patient is cold. Warm wraps are helpful for treating pulled muscles, bronchial spasms, and stomachaches caused by gastrointestinal infections.

They have a wonderfully relaxing effect on the body. A moist towel conducts heat much better than a dry hot water bottle.

The temperature of the liquid used for the wrap should be between 104 and 113 degrees Fahrenheit. Leave the wrap on for 3/4 of an hour to an hour. If it cools off too fast and makes the patient feel chilly, the wrap must be removed sooner.

Use warm wraps to help the body relax

Recipes

Ingredients Used for Warm Wraps
Hay flowers
- improve blood circulation and reduce cramping
- are recommended for pulled muscles and chronic bronchitis

▶ *This is how it's done:*
Heat a sachet with hay flowers over steam.

Chamomile
- relieves inflammation, promotes wound healing
- for infected wounds or acne

▶ *This is how it's done:*
Pour a quart of hot water over a handful of flowers.

Potato
- has a strong warming effect; relieves pain
- for pulled muscles and chronic bronchitis

▶ *This is how it's done:*
Boil potatoes and mash them. Spread the paste onto the middle third of a triple-sized towel. Fold the outer thirds of the towel over to cover the paste. Before applying the wrap face down, make sure that it's not too hot.

Ground mustard
- increases blood flow to the skin, fights bacteria and fungi
- for sore throats, chronic bronchitis, sinus infections, and liver and kidney ailments

▶ *This is how it's done:*
Dip the inner towel into warm water. Wring out any excess liquid. Spread two tablespoons of ground mustard seed evenly over the

middle third of the triple-sized towel. Never apply ground mustard directly to skin. Leave mustard wraps on the skin for no more than thirty minutes. Rinse the treated area. Ground mustard is a strong irritant and should therefore not be used on sensitive skin or for treating venous disorders. Do not use a ground mustard wrap on a child or adult who is too young or too ill to tell you it is too hot.

Onion
- stimulates the body's metabolism; reduces inflammation; disinfects, relieves pain, and acts as an expectorant
- useful for earaches, insect stings, colds, coughs, and urinary bladder infections

▶ *This is how it's done:*
Cut two to three onions into thin slices. Wrap them in a towel that's three times the size of the area to be treated. Put the wrap onto a screen placed over a pot of boiling water. Allow the rising steam to heat the onions. Before applying the wrap, slightly crush the sliced onions inside the cloth. To relieve an earache, place unheated onion slices into a small bag made of thin cloth and apply it to the affected ear.

Throat Wraps

Warm throat wraps are a very effective treatment for sore throats. Cold throat wraps reduce inflammation and are used to treat strep throat accompanied by fever and tonsilitis. They are also recommended for sinus infections and colds.

▶ *This is how it's done:*
- The inner towel used for a throat wrap should be about the width of a hand and long enough to be wrapped twice around the neck.
- For sore throats, ground mustard is helpful, as are potato paste, onion, or herbal decoctions.
- Cold throat wraps are prepared with cold water and vinegar, mineral clay, or yogurt.

Recipes

Chest Wraps

Cold chest wraps are excellent for all acute ailments of the respiratory tract. They improve circulation, act as an expectorant in cases of acute bronchitis, and relieve tickling in the throat. Symptoms of neurocirculatory asthenia, a condition also called "nervous heart" or "soldier's heart," such as rapid heart beat or minor arrhythmia (irregular heartbeat), can also be treated with cold chest wraps.

Chest wraps can even relieve asthma

Hot chest wraps are used primarily to relieve chronic bronchitis. They reduce bronchial spasms and act as an expectorant.

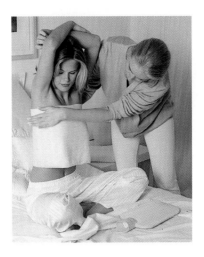 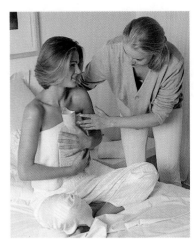

This is how you apply a hot chest wrap

Recipe

▶ *This is how it's done:*
A chest wrap envelops the entire rib cage and covers the area from the armpits down to below the arch of the ribs. You can add vinegar to cold water, herbs to warm water.

Abdominal Wraps

Not recommended for stomach or duodenal ulcers

Recipe

Warm abdominal wraps provide comfortable warmth and relax the abdominal organs. They relieve abdominal pain, gas, and diarrhea, and are used to treat urinary bladder infections.
▶ *This is how it's done:*
An abdominal wrap covers the area of the upper and lower abdomen. Use plain hot water, or add herbs.

Lumbar Wraps

Recipe

Cold wraps applied to the lumbar region aid intestinal function, relieve abdominal gas, and are helpful for treating ailments involving the liver or gallbladder. They can also be used in conjunction with conventional medical treatment for stomach and duodenal ulcers.
▶ *This is how it's done:*
Wraps applied to the lumbar region cover the area between the navel and the middle thigh. You can add salt or vinegar to the water.

Calf Wraps

Cold wraps applied to the calves reduce fever, relieve inflammation, firm tissues, and improve circulation in tired, aching legs. They

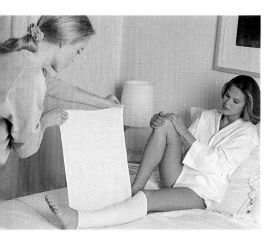
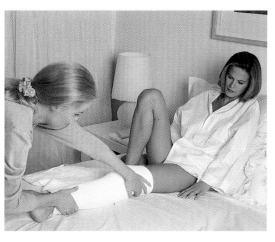

benefit people with varicose veins or phlebitis. Calf wraps also regulate blood circulation, have a calming effect, and promote sleep.

▶ *This is how it's done:*
A calf wrap covers the area of the leg between the hollow of the knee to the ankle. If you are using it to reduce a fever, the wrap should be changed every five minutes. When used to regulate venous and cardiovascular function, calf wraps can be left on for at least twenty minutes. Vinegar and salt are often added to the water.

This is how you apply a calf wrap

Packs

When treating ailments that affect smaller areas of the body, packs and compresses are the applications of choice. Various poultices can be used in combination with packs to relieve specific symptoms. Earaches, sinus infections, headaches, coughs, bronchitis, pulled muscles, and neuritis are among the ailments that can be treated most effectively with packs and compresses. Since they are applied to smaller areas, these applications are less stimulating than wraps. This makes them very appropriate for weak patients. Packs and compresses also require a shorter rest period following their application.

▶ *This is how it's done:*
Depending on the size of the area to be treated, you can either wrap the ingredients, such as boiled potatoes or onions, in a linen or cotton towel, or put them into a linen sachet. Place the pack or compress on the affected area. For ear compresses, a regular cloth handkerchief will work fine.

Recipe

Hay Flower Sachets

A hay flower sachet relieves pain and cramps and improves circulation. It can be placed on a painful joint or a pulled muscle in the neck or back. Hay flower sachets are also recommended for abdominal cramps, nausea, gas, constipation, and liver or kidney ailments.

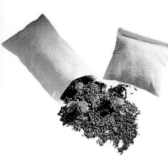

▶ *This is what you need:*
a hay flower sachet, a towel as a cover, a wool cloth, hot water

▶ *This is how it's done:*
- Fill a pot with water and cover it with a screen. Place the hay flower sachet on top. Boil the water and allow the rising steam to heat up the sachet until it's as hot as you can tolerate on your skin.
- Squeeze out any excess moisture and place the sachet on your skin. Cover it with a dry towel first, then add a wool cloth.
- Each hay flower sachet is used just once.

Not for use by people who have hay fever or allergies to hay

Compresses

Compresses are very easy to apply and do not require much time. Compresses are recommended for treating torn ligaments, bruises, sprains, pulled muscles, and wounds. A rest period after the treatment is beneficial, but not absolutely necessary.

Recipe

▶ *This is what you need:*
a wash cloth or small hand towel, a slightly larger towel, herbs such as chamomile, if desired

▶ *This is how it's done:*
Soak the wash cloth or small towel in cold water—or warm water if you're treating a pulled muscle—then wring it out. Fold it once and place it on the painful area. Cover everything with the larger towel. You can add various herbs, such as chamomile, to the water.

Baths, Affusions, and Washings

Aside from promoting relaxation, water applications provide stimuli that improve blood circulation and general health. Since emotional well-being and the immune system are closely linked, one of the benefits of water applications is better immune function.

Temperature

The stimulus provided by varying water temperatures is the most important aspect of Kneipp's hydrotherapy. Aside from wraps, this therapy includes baths and two other applications developed by Kneipp, washings and affusions.

- **Cold** applications improve blood circulation and are refreshing yet at the same time calming. They are appropriate only if the patient feels warm. After the treatment, the body needs to be warmed up immediately—either through exercise or by resting in a warm bed.
- **Warm** applications, such as warm baths, a series of baths of increasing temperature, or hot-moist wraps, improve blood circulation, speed up the body's metabolism, relax tense muscles, and improve local immune function. Worsening pain is a signal that warm applications are the wrong choice. They are also not recommended for people suffering from varicose veins, lymphatic edema, and impaired blood flow in the arteries.
- **Alternating cold and hot** baths have the strongest effect on the body. As a rule, the longer the body is immersed in cold water, and the lower the water temperature, the greater are the benefits to the immune system and to the entire organism.

Be careful if you have varicose veins, lymphatic edema, or poor circulation in the arteries

A thermometer will help you develop a feel for the right water temperature

Ingredients for Baths and Washings

Cold applications are usually done without adding any ingredients to the water. However, when an astringent or antibacterial effect is desired, or when the purpose of a washing or bath is to reduce swelling or itching, you can add apple cider vinegar to the cold water. For all warm applications, adding essential oils or herbs such as arnica, valerian, green tea (see page 29), hay flowers, chamomile (see page 100), lavender (see page 130), lemon balm, or rosemary is recommended. These ingredients enhance the prophylactic or healing effect of the treatment.

Baths

Full Baths

A *cold* full bath helps prevent colds and enhances the patient's general mood. It also stimulates and improves blood circulation. Stay in the bathtub for up to ten minutes, then exercise or rest in a warm bed.

In contrast, a *warm* full bath is relaxing and reduces pain. It is recommended for pulled muscles, stiff neck, and for various symptoms associated with osteoarthritis, lumbago, rheumatoid conditions, and gout. At the first sign of a cold, take a bath in warm water (about 104 degrees Fahrenheit) for up to twenty minutes.

Alternating between warm and cold temperatures is indicated for patients with circulatory problems for whom a warm bath by itself

For body and soul

would be too stimulating. Simply take a cold shower after a warm bath or—if you are very sensitive—do only a cold knee or arm affusion.

Arm Baths

An arm bath is done sitting down in front of a sink, or using a washtub especially designed for arm baths. The water has to cover the lower and half of the upper arm. Rest your elbows comfortably on the bottom of the sink or tub.

A comfortable body position is important during an arm bath

Cold arm baths help you get rid of tiredness, are refreshing, improve blood circulation, and have a calming effect.

▶ *This is how it's done:*
Immerse your arms for half a minute, then wipe off the water with your hands. Slowly swing your arms back and forth for about two minutes.

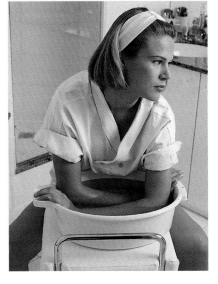

Patients with cardiovascular problems benefit most from arm baths that alternate between warm and cold water. These baths lower blood pressure, improve cardiovascular function and respiration, and help relieve tightness in the chest, dizziness, and osteoarthritis in the finger joints. Alternating warm and cold arm baths also help warm up chronically cold hands. For this type of application, you need two sinks or small tubs, one with cold, the other with warm water (95 to 100 degrees Fahrenheit).

▶ *This is how it's done:*
Immerse your arms first in warm water for five minutes, then in cold water for about fifteen to thirty minutes. Repeat once.

You need a sink or a small washtub for immersing the arms

Foot Baths

For foot baths, you need a bucket or a Kneipp foot tub filled with enough water to cover your legs up to the knees.

Cold foot baths are recommended if you have difficulty falling asleep. They are also helpful in treating various ailments affecting the legs, such as loss of tone in the walls of veins, tired legs after prolonged sitting or walking, or bruises on the ankle or foot.

Recommended for cardiovascular ailments and cold hands

▶ *This is how it's done:*
Immerse your legs for a minute, then wipe off the water with your hands. Dry the bottom of your feet and put on a pair of long cotton socks. Rest.

Ask your doctor if this kind of application is suitable for you

● *Warm* foot baths improve blood circulation and have a relaxing effect on the lower abdominal organs. (They are also helpful for menstrual problems or urinary bladder infections.) This type of application is recommended for treating slow-healing wounds and ulcers in the lower leg area. However, warm foot baths should not be used if there is any infection on the foot or lower leg.

▶ *This is how it's done:*
The legs stay immersed in water for up to five minutes (if you have varicose veins, the water should come up only to your ankles and be no warmer than 91 degrees Fahrenheit).

● *Alternating warm and cold* foot baths stabilize circulatory function, train the body to adjust to changes in temperature, are beneficial at the first signs of a cold, relieve headaches, and promote sleep. If you have ulcers on your lower legs or varicose veins that are not infected, you can use this type of application, provided that the water temperature does not exceed 91 degrees Fahrenheit. To be safe, ask your doctor first! The easiest way to do alternating warm and cold foot baths is to place two buckets in your bathtub. One bucket is filled with cold, the other with warm water of about 99 degrees Fahrenheit (if you have varicose veins, the water should come up only to your ankles and be no warmer than 91 degrees Fahrenheit).

+ See a doctor

▶ *This is how it's done:*
Sitting on the rim of the bathtub, first immerse your legs in warm water for five minutes, then in cold water for twenty minutes. Repeat once. Instead of using a bucket with cold water, you can rinse your legs with cold water from a hose.

Not for patients with venous infections, either on the surface or deeper inside the legs

Treading Water

Treading water is refreshing, improves blood circulation, regulates body temperature, calms the nervous system, reduces susceptibility to colds and infections, and strengthens the walls of the veins in the legs. Treading water also relieves stress. If you are hypersensitive to atmospheric changes and experience confusion, exhaustion, or a feeling of pressure in the head as a result of this condition, this type of application may be able to help you. People who tread water in the evening report better sleep. Treading water can be done at home in your bathtub or you can take a walk stork-fashion in wet grass or in snow!

Important: Always make sure that your legs are warm before you start treading water. This application is not recommended if you have an acute urinary tract infection, poor blood circulation, or leg cramps.

Important!

▶ *This is how it's done:*
Fill the bathtub with cold water. Like a stork (i.e., lifting each leg entirely out of the water with each step), wade through the water for thirty seconds to a minute. Wipe off the water with your hands, put on a pair of long cotton socks or stockings, and either walk around a warm room until your feet are warm, or immediately warm them up in bed.

Affusions

Cold or alternating warm and cold affusions improve cardiovascular function, the body's ability to adjust to changes in temperature, and respiration. For an affusion to be as effective as possible, the stream of water has to form a solid sheet that gently envelops the limb or part of the body being treated. Many showerheads have settings that allow you to do this. Each affusion can be done either cold, warm, alternating warm and cold, or hot. It should last 1 1/2 to 4 minutes, depending on the area of application and the sensitivity of the patient. As a rule, the water is poured from the outside towards the center of the body.

Important!

Important: Patients who are elderly, suffer from poor circulation, or have a sensitive nervous system should always rest for fifteen minutes after affusions to large areas of the body.

Orthopedic supply stores may sell special attachments for your showerhead

Facial Affusions

Cold facial affusions are mentally and physically refreshing, improve respiration and blood flow to the skin, and are helpful for various ailments that affect the head, such as headaches, migraines, dizziness, vertigo, or impaired vision or hearing.

Alternating warm and cold affusions are also very beneficial. You first use warm water for about fifteen seconds, then cold water for five seconds. Repeat once.

▶ *This is how it's done:*
Starting with the forehead and moving clockwise, pour a gentle stream of water over your face. Breathe through your mouth. Don't hold your breath!

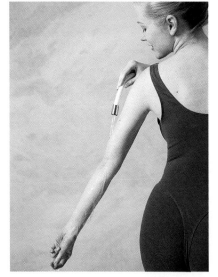

Arm Affusions

Cold arm affusions are refreshing, cause you to breathe deeper, and improve blood circulation. They make your heartbeat slightly stronger, which is desirable.

Alternating cold and warm affusions normalize low blood pressure and have a stimulating and refreshing effect when you're exhausted or find it hard to concentrate. Alternate thirty seconds of warm and fifteen seconds of cold water. Repeat once or twice.

The stream of water should form a sheet that envelops the limb or body

▶ *This is how it's done:*
Beginning at the back of your right hand, move the stream of water upwards until you reach the shoulder. Keep it there for a while, then move downward along the inner arm. Repeat on the left arm.

Knee Affusions

Cold knee affusions have a calming effect and are used to treat insomnia. They strengthen the blood vessels and bring relief for heavy, aching legs and feet.

Alternating warm and cold knee affusions are mainly used for arthritic knee conditions. Both lower legs are treated first with warm water for half a minute, then with cold water for ten seconds. Repeat once.

▶ *This is how it's done:*
Start at the right foot. Move the stream of water back and forth along the sole from heel to toes two or three times, then up along the outside of the lower leg to about a hand's breadth above the knee. Keep it there for a while, then move downward along the inner leg to the heel. Repeat on the left foot.

A knee affusion can be extended to include the thigh and lower abdomen

Thigh Affusions

When a knee affusion is extended upwards to the buttocks, it becomes a thigh affusion. This type of application is intended to treat ailments affecting the thighs, hip joints and buttocks, such as osteoarthritis of the hip joints, sciatica, or rheumatoid conditions affecting the muscles.

Abdominal Affusions

A thigh affusion that continues upward toward the bottom of the rib cage is called an abdominal affusion. It affects the entire organism by relaxing the body and improving metabolic function and digestion. Abdominal affusions relieve minor constipation, chronic abdominal distension, gastritis, stomach ulcers, irritable bowel syndrome in the colon, and general pain and cramping in the abdomen or the muscles of the lower back. They are also used to treat disorders involving the uterus, the kidneys, and the urinary bladder.

Back Affusions

Alternating warm and cold back affusions are recommended for ailments affecting the spine. They relieve pain due to damaged discs or pulled muscles. If you suffer from a spinal disorder, you need to be careful with cold water. *Warm* affusions are generally preferable for such conditions.

▶ *This is how it's done:*
Start at the right foot and move the stream of water upward until you reach the buttocks. Move down the inner leg and repeat the procedure on the left leg. Now move from the right hand along the arm to the shoulder blade. Stay there for a few seconds, then proceed down the back until you reach the buttocks. Repeat on the left side.

Always start on the right side, then proceed to the left

Full Body Affusions

When a back affusion is expanded to include the chest and stomach, it becomes a full body affusion. This application is best done with *alternating warm and cold* water. Use warm water for a minute, then switch to cold for twenty seconds. Repeat once. Or do a *warm* full body affusion followed by a cold affusion limited to the knees.

▶ *This is how it's done:*
Move the stream of water along the outside of the right leg from the foot up to the hip. Keep it there for a few seconds, moving back and forth between the buttocks and the groin so that the water is spread evenly over the entire leg. Do the same on the left side. Next, move on to the arms. Starting at the right hand, move upwards along your arm to your shoulder. Stay there for a few seconds and let the water flow over your chest and back. Repeat on the left side.

Washings

Regular washings are especially effective for strengthening the body's immune system and for improving blood circulation. When limited to specific parts of the body, they provide only a mild stimulus, making them very suitable even for patients who have been seriously weakened by illness. A full body or partial washing in the morning starts the day well and can be used to complement morning gymnastics. If you wake up in the middle of the night and can't go back to sleep, a partial washing can be of help. It should be done quickly, however, and the water should be spread evenly over the body. This is more important than moving the terry cloth mitten along the body exactly as described.

▶ *This is what you need:*
a terry cloth mitten, apple cider vinegar or salt if desired

▶ *This is how it's done:*
- Dip the terry cloth mitten into cold water (54 to 61 degrees Fahrenheit). Wring it out until it no longer drips. If you are sensitive to cold temperatures, you may want to start with 68-degree water and gradually lower the temperature with each subsequent washing. In small children, wash only the arms using water temperatures between 86 to 95 degrees Fahrenheit. Apply even, gentle pressure as you wash the different areas of the body.
- Do not dry yourself off afterwards. Put your pajamas back on and rest in a warm bed until the body is thoroughly warm throughout.
- To increase the stimulus provided by the water, you can add apple cider vinegar or salt: use about one part vinegar to two parts water, or two tablespoons of sea salt for each half-quart of water (allow the salt to dissolve before you start the washing).

Upper Body Washing

A series of washings is recommended at the first signs of a cold. Their purpose is to make you sweat. At twenty- to thirty-minute intervals, repeat the following procedure several times: Wash your upper body, then warm up immediately in a warm bed. As an added benefit, serial washings are a quick and effective way to help the body rid itself of toxins. If you want to improve your body's resistance to infection, try daily upper body washings at bedtime for a few weeks in the fall.

For upper respiratory colds and for reducing susceptibility to infections

▶ *This is how it's done:*
Wash the right arm first, then the neck, chest, and stomach area, then the left arm, and finally the back.

Washings of the Abdomen and Legs

Cold washings of the legs or of the entire body below the waist create a good diversion and have a calming effect, making them a excellent treatment for insomnia. After the body is washed and warmed up, a restful sleep often follows quickly. This kind of application is also beneficial for people who suffer from poor blood circulation in the morning, who have varicose veins, cold feet, or constipation, or whose nervous system is overstimulated.

This application will help you sleep

▶ *This is how it's done:*
Start the washing on the instep of your right foot. Move up along the outer leg until you reach the pelvis, then wash the front of the leg down to the foot. Move up once more along the inner leg to the groin. Repeat on the left leg. Now wash the buttocks and the abdominal area with circular, clockwise motions.

Full Body Washings

When doing this type of washing, speed is essential so that the body can get warmed up again as quickly as possible.

▶ *This is how it's done:*
Start at the back of the right hand. Wash the outside of the arm up to the shoulder, then down along the inner arm. Do the same to the left arm. Now wash the chest with horizontal motions, then the abdomen with vertical motions. Next, proceed along the outside of the right leg down to the foot, then back up along the inner leg to the groin. Repeat on the left side. Finally, wash the back from the neck down to the buttocks.

Effective Remedies for Specific Ailments

Symptoms	Remedy	Application	Page
General health			
Physical and mental exhaustion during or after periods of over-exertion, illness, exposure to environmental toxins or radiation, general weakness and reduced stamina, seasonal fatigue	Apple cider vinegar	Cure with apple cider vinegar-honey drink	18
	Echinacea	Cure with tincture	113
	Garlic	Take fresh garlic or a garlic supplement	27
	Ginseng	Take powder or capsules	123
	Green tea	Drink regularly	34
	Honey	Cure with plain honey	45
	Hydrotherapy	Cold or warm baths	163
	Stinging nettle	Cure with fresh juice	147
Allergy			
General	Black cumin	Take oil or capsules	94
	Honey	Cure with plain honey	47
Allergic asthma	Black cumin	Take oil or capsules, inhale with seeds and oil	94
	Chest wraps	Cold with apple cider vinegar	159
	Honey	Cure with plain honey	47
Hay fever	Black cumin	Take oil or capsules; inhale with seeds and oil	93
Blood vessels			
Arteriosclerosis	Garlic	Take fresh garlic or a supplement	27
	Ginseng	Take powder or capsules	124
	Green tea	Drink regularly	32
	Kefir/Kombucha	Drink daily	52
	Mistletoe	Cure with mistletoe tea	137
	Sauerkraut	Eat regularly	72
Circulatory problems	Garlic	Take fresh garlic or a supplement	27
	Ginkgo	Take a ginkgo supplement	120
	Wine	Drink regularly as a prophylactic	74
	Wraps	Cold wraps with apple cider vinegar	157
Hemorrhoids	Apple cider vinegar	Lukewarm sitz bath	22
Varicose veins	Apple cider vinegar	Cold calf wraps, foot baths, washings	157
	Hydrotherapy	Cold affusions, washings	166
	Wraps	Cold, with apple cider vinegar, yogurt, or salt	157
Phlebitis	Calf wraps	Cold, with apple cider vinegar or yogurt	160
	Hydrotherapy	Cold affusions, washings	166
Cancer			
In conjunction with conventional treatment	Ginseng	Take powder or extract	125
	Mistletoe	To be administered only by a qualified health practitioner	137
Prevention	Ginseng	A cure with powder or extract	125
	Green tea	Drink regularly	34
	Sauerkraut	Eat regularly to prevent duodenal cancer	72

Effective Remedies for Specific Ailments

Symptoms	Remedy	Application	Page
Cardiovascular disorders			
High blood pressure	Garlic	Take fresh garlic or a garlic supplement	27
	Honey	Take regularly, either plain or dissolved in water	44
	Mistletoe	Cure with mistletoe tea	137
Low blood pressure,	Arm bath	Alternating warm/cold, with essential oils	164
circulatory problems	Calf wrap	Cold, with apple cider vinegar	160
	Ginseng	Take powder or extract	124
	Lavender	Baths	133
	Water	Cold baths, affusions, washings	162
Myocardial insufficiency	Hawthorn	Drink hawthorn tea or take a supplement	127
(decreased heart function)	Honey	Take regularly, either plain or dissolved in tea	46
	Hawthorn	Tea from herbal mixture	129
Neurocirculatory asthenia	Honey	Take plain or dissolved in tea	46
(nervous heart)	Mistletoe	Cure with mistletoe tea	137
Children's ailments			
Bed wetting	St. John's wort	Drink tea and massage oil onto abdomen and inner thighs	144
Failure to thrive	Honey	Cure with honey taken plain or dissolved in tea	48
Poor concentration, hyperactivity	Honey	Cure with honey taken plain or dissolved in tea	48
Stomachache	Chamomile	Drink tea, warm stomach wrap	105
	St. John's wort	Warm stomach wrap; massage stomach area with oil; drink tea	144
	Stomach wrap	Warm, with hay flowers, chamomile, or St. John's wort	158
Teething	Chamomile	Let granules dissolve in the mouth	105
Ears			
Earache	Wrap	With onion	159
Ringing in the ears	Ginkgo	Take a ginkgo supplement	120
	Hydrotherapy	Cold facial affusion	166
Eyes			
Conjunctivitis	Echinacea	Take tincture; apply packs with paste or ointment	113
Sties	Echinacea	Take tincture; apply packs with paste or ointment	113

Effective Remedies for Specific Ailments

Symptoms	Remedy	Application	Page
Gastrointestinal disorders			
Abdominal gas	Apple cider vinegar	Apple cider vinegar-honey drink	22
	Black cumin	Take seeds, oil, or capsules; drink tea made from seeds	95
	Chamomile	Drink tea	103
	Garlic	Take fresh garlic or a supplement	28
	Lavender	Drink tea	133
	Onion	Eat fresh or take onion syrup	58
	St. John's wort	Drink tea	144
	Wraps	Warm, with chamomile or St. John's wort	158
Constipation	Abdominal wraps	Warm, with apple cider vinegar, chamomile, potato, St. John's wort	160
	Apple cider vinegar	Warm stomach wraps; apple cider vinegar-honey drink	22
	Black cumin	Take seeds, oil, or capsules; drink cumin seed tea; abdominal wraps	95
	Honey	Take plain or in laxative tea	47
	Hydrotherapy	Cold affusions, washings	166
	Onion	Eat fresh, or take onion syrup	58
	Sauerkraut	Drink juice, eat sauerkraut	72
	Stomach wraps	Warm, with apple cider vinegar, chamomile, potato, St. John's wort	158
Diarrhea, general	Apple cider vinegar	Take diluted in uncarbonated mineral water	22
	Black cumin	Take seeds, oil, or capsules; drink cumin seed tea	95
	Green tea	Drink	35
	St. John's wort	Drink tea; warm wraps with oil	144
	Wraps	Warm, with chamomile, potato, or St. John's wort	158
–caused by bacteria	Garlic	Take garlic in high doses	28
	Honey	Take plain	47
	Wraps	Warm, with chamomile, potato, St. John's wort	158
Gallbladder ailments	Vegetable oils	Take olive oil or other cold-pressed vegetable oils	66
Gastritis	Chamomile	Drink tea; rolling cure	104
	St. John's wort	Take tea or oil; warm packs	144
	Vegetable oils	Take olive or other nutritionally valuable vegetable oils	66

Effective Remedies for Specific Ailments

Symptoms	Remedy	Application	Page
Gastrointestinal disorders (continued)			
Irritable bowel syndrome, nervous indigestion	Chamomile	Drink tea	104
	Garlic	Take fresh, powder or tablets	28
	Green tea	Drink regularly instead of coffee	35
	Honey	Take plain or dissolved in digestive tea	47
	Kefir/Kombucha	Drink daily	54
	Lavender	Drink tea	133
	Sauerkraut	Drink sauerkraut or cabbage juice	72
	Wraps	Warm, with chamomile, potato, or St. John's wort	158
Loss of appetite	Green tea	Drink before each meal	35
	Honey	Take plain	47
	Onion	Eat raw or take onion syrup	58
Nausea, vomiting	Black cumin	Take seeds, oil, or capsules; drink cumin seed tea	95
	Chamomile	Drink tea	104
	Packs	Warm hay flower sachet	162
	St. John's wort	Take oil or drink tea	144
Stomachaches	Chamomile	Drink tea; warm stomach wraps	104
	Packs	Warm hay flower sachet	162
	St. John's wort	Warm stomach packs; massage stomach with oil; drink tea	144
Infections and immune system disorders			
Bronchitis	Apple cider vinegar	Inhale; cold or warm chest wraps; drink with honey	20
	Arm bath	Increasingly warmer temperature, add essential oil to water	164
	Black cumin	Take oil or capsules; inhale with seeds or oil	94
	Chamomile	Drink tea; inhale	104
	Chest wraps	Cold, with apple cider vinegar or yogurt; warm, with chamomile, mustard seed, onion, or potato	157
	Echinacea	Take tincture	114
	Garlic	Take garlic juice	28
	Green tea	Drink; inhale	35
	Honey	Cure with plain honey or honey dissolved in bronchial tea	47
	Onion	Inhale; eat raw or take onion syrup	59
Cold, flu	Apple cider vinegar	Inhale; drink with honey	20
	Black cumin	Take oil or capsules	94
	Chamomile	Drink tea; inhale	104
	Echinacea	Drink tea or take tincture	114
	Green tea	Drink; inhale	35
	Honey	Take plain or dissolved in tea for colds	47

Effective Remedies for Specific Ailments

Symptoms	Remedy	Application	Page
Infections and immune system disorders (continued)			
Cough	Apple cider vinegar	Inhale; drink with honey	20
	Arm bath	Increasingly warm, with essential oil as an additive	164
	Chamomile	Drink tea; inhale	104
	Chest wraps	Cold, with apple cider vinegar; warm, with bee's wax, chest balm, or potato	159
	Echinacea	Drink tea or take tincture	114
	Garlic	Take garlic juice	28
	Onion	Drink hot onion milk	59
Fever	Calf wrap	Cold	160
	Foot bath	For chills, increasingly warm	165
	Washings	Cold	168
Immune deficiency	Aloe vera	Cure with aloe juice	89
	Apple cider vinegar	Cold wraps; washings; apple cider vinegar-honey drink	157
	Black cumin	Take oil or capsules	94
	Chest wraps	Warm with apple cider vinegar or salt	159
	Echinacea	Cure with echinacea tincture	113
	Foot bath	Increasingly warm	165
	Ginseng	Cure with powder or extract	124
	Green tea	Drink regularly	34
	Honey	Cure with plain honey	47
	Washings	Cool, with essential oil	168
Shingles	Echinacea	Wrap with paste or diluted tincture; take tincture	114
	Packs	With cabbage leaves	71
	St. John's wort	Dab with oil; drink tea, or take a St. John's wort supplement	144
	Apple cider vinegar	Inhale; damp-hot throat wraps; apple cider vinegar-honey drink	158
Sore throat	Chamomile	Gargle with tea	104
	Echinacea	Gargle with diluted tincture	114
	Green tea	Gargle with strong tea	35
	Honey	Take plain, or drink diluted in tea, milk, or lemon	47
	Throat wraps	Warm or cold, with apple cider vinegar, yogurt, or mustard seed	159
Kidney and Bladder			
Bladder irritation	Vegetable oil	Take pumpkin seed oil regularly	66
	Stinging nettle	Drink tea	149
Small kidney stones	Apple cider vinegar	Apple cider vinegar-honey drink	20

Effective Remedies for Specific Ailments

Symptoms	Remedy	Application	Page
Kidney and Bladder (continued)			
Urinary bladder infection	Echinacea	Take tincture	114
	Honey	Take plain or dissolved in tea	47
	Onion	Warm onion pack	59
	Stinging nettle	Drink tea	149
Men's ailments			
Enlarged prostate	Stinging nettle	Take stinging nettle tincture or supplement	149
Impotence	Vegetable oil	Take pumpkin seed oil regularly	66
	Ginseng	Cure with powder or extract	125
Metabolism			
Overweight	Apple cider vinegar	Cure with apple cider vinegar-honey drink	18
	Sauerkraut	Cure with sauerkraut	71
Detoxification	Apple cider vinegar	Cure with apple cider vinegar-honey drink	18
	Green tea	Drink regularly instead of coffee or black tea	34
	Honey	Take plain or dissolved in tea	47
	Kefir/Kombucha	Drink daily	54
Elevated lipid levels in the blood	Evening primrose	Take evening primrose oil capsules	117
	Garlic	Eat fresh or take a supplement	28
	Ginseng	Take powder or extract	124
	Vegetable oils	Use cold-pressed vegetable oils	63
	Wine	Drink regularly for prevention	74
Mouth and teeth			
Bad breath	Apple cider vinegar	Gargle with diluted apple cider vinegar	20
	Green tea	Rinse and gargle with tea	35
Cavities	Green tea	Rinse; drink tea for prevention	35
Cold sores	Echinacea	Apply ointment; dab with tincture	114
	St. John's wort	Dab affected area with oil	144
Gingivitis or inflammation of the mucous membranes of the mouth	Apple cider vinegar	Rinse mouth, dab on gums	20
	Calendula	Rinse or gargle with tea	99
	Chamomile	Rinse with strong tea	105
	Echinacea	Gargle with diluted tincture	114
	Green tea	Rinse with strong tea	35
Nervous system and brain			
Alzheimer's disease	Ginkgo	Take a ginkgo supplement	120
Depression	Ginseng	Take powder or extract	125
	Hydrotherapy	Cold baths, affusions, washings	163
	Packs	Warm hay flower sachet	162
	St. John's wort	Drink tea or take a supplement	142
Dizziness	Ginkgo	Take a ginkgo supplement	120
	Hydrotherapy	Cold facial affusion	166

Effective Remedies for Specific Ailments

Symptoms	Remedy	Application	Page
Nervous System and Brain (continued)			
Headache, migraine	Apple cider vinegar	Apple cider vinegar-honey drink; cold compress on the forehead	20
	Arm bath	Warm, with essential oil added	164
	Compresses, packs	Cold, with yogurt; warm, with apple cider vinegar, essential oil, or potato	161
	Foot bath	Increasingly warm	165
	Garlic	Take fresh garlic or a supplement	27
	Hydrotherapy	Cold facial affusion	166
Insomnia	Calf wrap	Cold or warm, with apple cider vinegar, chamomile, lavender, or St. John's wort	160
	Garlic	Take fresh garlic, garlic powder, or tablets	27
	Honey	Dissolve in tea for insomnia	46
	Hydrotherapy	Cold, warm, or alternating cold/warm baths, cold washings	163
	Lavender	Drink tea; baths; herbal sachets	133
	Packs	Warm hay flower sachet	162
	St. Johns's wort	Drink tea or take as a supplement	143
Memory loss	Ginkgo	Take a ginkgo supplement	120
	Honey	Take plain or dissolved in tea	46
Mental exhaustion	Ginseng	Take ginseng powder or extract	123
	Honey	Take plain or dissolved in tea	45
	Hydrotherapy	Cold baths, affusions, washings	162
	St. John's wort	Drink tea or take a supplement	142
Nervousness	Garlic	Take fresh or as a supplement	27
	Honey	Take plain or dissolved in a calming tea; abdominal wrap	46
	Lavender	Drink tea; baths	132
	Packs	Warm hay flower sachet	162
	St. John's wort	Drink tea or take a supplement	142
Neuralgia	Packs	Warm hay flower sachet	162
	St. John's wort	Drink tea or take a supplement; warm compresses with oil	144
Poor concentration	Honey	Take plain or dissolved in tea	46
	St. John's wort	Drink tea or take a supplement	142
Muscles, Bones, and Joints			
Back pain	Compresses	Cold, with apple cider vinegar or yogurt; warm, with apple cider vinegar, essential oil, potato, or St. John's wort	161
	Hydrotherapy	Warm/cold or warm affusions	166
	Packs	Warm hay flower sachet	162
	St. John's wort	Warm compresses with oil	144

Effective Remedies for Specific Ailments

Symptoms	Remedy	Application	Page
Muscles, Bones, and Joints (continued)			
Gout	Green tea	Drink regularly as a prophylactic	34
	Wraps	Warm or cold, with cabbage leaves	155
Joint pain, arthritis	Apple cider vinegar	Apple cider vinegar-honey drink	21
	Stinging nettle	Drink tea; take fruit or use them for a pack; rub in nettle spirit	149
Muscle pain, pulled muscles	St. John's wort	Massage, warm wrap with oil	144
	Wraps	Warm, with chamomile, hay flowers, potato, St. John's wort oil	158
Osteoarthritis	Hydrotherapy	Cold affusions, baths	162
	Mistletoe	Cure with mistletoe tea; injections	137
	Packs	Warm hay flower sachet	162
Rheumatoid disorders	Apple cider vinegar	Cold or warm wraps; apple cider vinegar-honey drink	21
	Hydrotherapy	Cold affusions, washings	162
	Packs, wraps	Cold, with yogurt; warm, with cabbage leaves, hay flower sachet, onion, or potato	157
	Stinging nettle	Drink tea; take fruit or use them as a poultice; rub in nettle spirit	149
Skin and Hair			
Acne, very oily, blemished skin	Aloe vera	Apply gel, facial mask	89
	Apple cider vinegar	Facial steam bath; apple cider vinegar-honey drink	23
	Baths	Warm, with chamomile or St. John's wort	163
	Black cumin	Warm facial compresses with tea; take oil or capsules; steam bath with seeds or oil	95
	Calendula	Facial steam bath, baths	98
	Chamomile	Steam bath or compresses with tea	105
	Honey	Cosmetic preparations	48
	Packs	With apple cider vinegar, mineral-rich clay, yogurt	161
	St. John's wort	Facial bath; dab individual pimples	141
	Steam bath	With apple cider vinegar, chamomile, St. John's wort	163
	Stinging nettle	Cure with stinging nettle tea	149
Dry skin	Black cumin	Take oil or capsules; massage oil into cracked skin	95
	Chamomile	Rub in oil; apply oil or ointment to cracked skin	105
	Evening primrose	Take capsules containing oil	117
	Green tea	Wash with it; drink regularly	35
	Vegetable oil	Use as massage or bath oil	67

Effective Remedies for Specific Ailments

Symptoms	Remedy	Application	Page
Skin and Hair (continued)			
Eczema	Black cumin	Take oil or capsules; apply oil to affected areas	95
	Calendula	Compresses; apply ointment	99
	Green tea	Wash with it; baths	35
Fungal skin infection	Apple cider vinegar	Massage into affected areas	23
	Black cumin	Take oil or capsules; apply oil to affected areas	95
Hair loss, hair care	Apple cider vinegar	Take diluted with water; rinse	23
	Black cumin	Take oil or capsules	95
	Packs	With cabbage leaves	161
	Stinging nettle	Rinse with decoction; massage into the scalp	149
Insect stings	Apple cider vinegar	Cold compresses	23
	Echinacea	Apply ointment	112
	Onion	Apply a slice of raw onion	59
Neurodermatitis	Black cumin	Take oil or capsules; massage in undiluted oil	95
	Evening primrose	Take capsules containing oil; apply undiluted oil to affected areas	117
Over-processed hair	Vegetable oil	Massage almond, wheat germ, or corn oil into hair	67
Skin infection, bacterial	Apple cider vinegar	Take diluted with water; compresses	23
	Calendula	Compresses with tea or ointment	98
	Chamomile	Compresses with tea	105
	Compress	Warm, with calendula, chamomile, or St. John's wort	162
	Echinacea	Dab on ointment; compress with paste or diluted tincture	112
	Honey	Apply to infected area	48
Stressed, tired-looking skin	Apple cider vinegar	Take diluted with water; baths, packs	23
	Green tea	Washings; drink regularly	35
	Washings	Cool, with essential oils	168
Sunburn, minor burns	Aloe vera	Apply commercially available gel or fresh gel from a leaf	89
	Apple cider vinegar	Compresses, lukewarm baths	23
	Echinacea	Apply ointment	112
	Green tea	Drink; use for packs	35
	Packs	With cabbage leaves, yogurt	163
	St. John's wort	Apply oil	143
Ulcer	Calendula	Warm wraps, compresses with tea or ointment	99

Effective Remedies for Specific Ailments

Symptoms	Remedy	Application	Page
Skin and Hair (continued)			
Wounds	Aloe vera	Apply commercially available gel or fresh gel from a leaf	89
	Apple cider vinegar	Take diluted with water; dab on wound	23
	Calendula	Warm wraps; compresses with tea or ointment	98
	Chamomile	Compress with strong tea	105
	Compresses	Warm, with calendula, chamomile, or St. John's wort	162
	Echinacea	Apply compresses with tincture or ointment	114
	Honey	Apply a thick layer to closed wounds	47
	St. John's wort	Apply compresses, oil	143
	White cabbage	Apply strips of leaves	72
Women's ailments			
Irregular periods	Chaste tree	Take supplement	108
Menopausal problems	Ginseng	Take powder or extract	124
Morning sickness	Apple cider vinegar	Apple cider vinegar-honey drink	21
PMS	Apple cider vinegar	Apple cider vinegar-honey drink	21
	Chaste tree	Take supplement	108
	Evening primrose	Take capsules containing oil	117
Pregnancy, birth	Honey	Take plain regularly; infusion	45
Vaginal discharge	Apple cider vinegar	Douche with diluted apple cider vinegar	22
Vaginal yeast infection	Echinacea	Take tincture	114

Resource Directory

The purpose of this book is to make it easy for you to use home remedies and herbs at all levels. Most of all, we want you to have access to these remedies whenever you need them. For this reason, we have included brief answers to questions that may come up as you use the various remedies. A list of addresses and related books is added to help you find practitioners, organizations, sources for products, and additional information on certain topics.

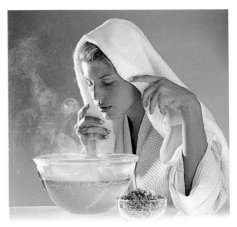

Inhaling with chamomile relieves colds

Answers to Frequently Asked Questions

Remedies from Your Kitchen
Many people experience abdominal gas and discomfort after eating sauerkraut. How can this be prevented?

▶ Heat the sauerkraut first without using any fat. Add caraway seeds, fennel, juniper berries, or a little honey. Sausages, meat, lard, or bacon are added only at the very end. If this does not take care of the problem, try the following: Chew some caraway seeds, or drink caraway tea. By the way: If you regularly eat sauerkraut or other vegetables of the cabbage family, your digestive system will get used to this type of food and you won't experience abdominal gas discomfort anymore.

What is the difference between flower honey and tree honey?

▶ Both types of honey are made from sugary liquids. As far as their source is concerned, these liquids do not have very much in common. As the name implies, flower honey is made from nectar produced by flowers. Tree honey is predigested honey dew, a substance secreted by tree-dwelling insects, such as lice, that live off their host's leaves or needles.

How do you preserve culinary herbs?

▶ The most commonly used method for preserving herbs is to hang them up to dry in an airy, shaded place immediately after harvesting. You can also freeze herbs, either finely chopped in ice cube trays, or whole, wrapped in aluminum foil. A third method is to preserve them in salt and olive oil, in oil, or in vinegar.

What is the difference between black and green tea?

▶ Both varieties of tea are made from the leaves of the same plant. After the harvest, leaves for black tea undergo a fermenting process catalyzed by their own enzymes. This turns them reddish-brown first, then black after they are dried. The process allows the body to absorb the caffeine in black tea more quickly, thus making it more stimulating than green tea. However, fermentation sacrifices some of the ingredients that are retained in green tea. Black tea is therefore little more than a consumer beverage. It's only marginally effective in relieving minor diarrhea. Black tea used to be grown mainly in the British colonies. Green tea is superior to black tea.

How can you tell if a vegetable oil has much nutritional value?

▶ Most of its valuable active ingredients, such as vitamins, flavonoids, and lecithin, as well as its aromatic compounds, are preserved only if the oil has been cold-pressed. Cold-pressed olive oil is labeled *extra virgin* or *virgin*. Refined oils have been heated to high temperatures and produced with chemical solvents. They contain fewer valuable ingredients, but have a longer shelf life. Unlike cold-pressed oils, refined oils do not contain unhealthy chemical substances after being heated. Rancid oil should not be used. It also contains substances that can be harmful to the body.

Resource Directory

Herbs

How long can you store dried herbs?

▶ When stored in a dark, dry place, flowers, leaves and roots retain their quality for about a year. After that, some active ingredients are destroyed and the herb loses more and more of its effectiveness. For this reason, harvest or buy only as much herbs as you are likely to use within one year.

Why can't you simply pour hot water over certain herbs to brew a tea?

▶ Plants that are rich in mucilage (e.g., European marsh mallow and holly-hock) require steeping overnight in cold water to ensure that the mucilage is not destroyed. The same is true for plants that contain large amounts of tannins (such as bearberry leaves and valerian). Cold water extraction results in a less bitter tea. Another method is to pour cold water over the herb and then simmer it for about five minutes over low heat in a ceramic pot. Remove it from the burner and let it steep for another five minutes; then strain it. This method is used primarily for roots and bark.

What are the potential side effects of herbs?

▶ Every medicine has the potential to cause unwanted side effects or interactions with other medicines. The same is true for herbs, although side effects happen less often, and when they occur, they are usually milder. When an herbal remedy affects such delicately balanced systems as the hormonal or immune system, it can have effects that are similar to that of a synthetic chemical substance. Very potent or very toxic compounds present in herbs can also cause problems, depending on the dosage and the sensitivity of the patient. It is also a fact that certain people experience allergic reactions to "completely harmless" plants.

Hydrotherapy

How do cold wraps work?

▶ Cold wraps first cause the peripheral blood vessels to constrict in order to protect the body from losing too much heat. As soon as the cold stimulus diminishes, a lot of warm, nutrient- and oxygen-rich blood flows to the affected area to restore the temporarily reduced supply. The rate of metabolic function in the area is increased considerably, as are respiration and lymphatic function. Via the nerves, the inner organs are also stimulated.

When should you use cold wraps, and when are warm wraps recommended?

▶ Colds wraps are used for acute conditions. They relieve inflammation and pain, stimulate metabolic function, and mobilize the body's defenses against disease. The organism has to expend energy to generate heat. When patients are already weakened due to illness, they should conserve energy. In this case, warm wraps are preferable. They provide warmth and support immune function rather than merely activating it. If the body part to be treated is cold, it must be warmed up with a warm wrap or a hot water bottle first. Warm wraps are not recommended if the patient is running a fever. Whether a wrap should be warm or cold depends mainly on the subjective feeling of the patient. A wrap should never feel uncomfortable. When the patient is a child, the stimuli provided by the wrap should be mild: cold wraps should not be too cold, hot wraps should merely be warm.

What is the difference between a wrap, a pack, and a compress?

▶ A pack is merely placed on the affected area, while a wrap, as the name implies, is wrapped around the entire body part being treated. An example of a pack is the hay flower sachet, which is placed on a painful joint, a pulled muscle, or on an uncomfortable stomach. Compresses are quick and easy to apply. All you need to do is dip a small hand towel in water and place it on a sports injury or wound.

General

What should I look for when choosing a health care practitioner?

▶ Good health care practitioners who use herbs and natural remedies—whether they practice conventional or alternative medicine—should first conduct a thorough interview (i.e., collect information about previous diagnoses and treatments, the patient's life style, work conditions, and diet). For a medical diagnosis, see a licensed physician. They should examine the patient thoroughly, set a goal for the treatment, and come up with a treatment plan that establishes a time after which the success of the treatment is to be evaluated. They inform the patient of the potential risks of the proposed treatment, are clear about their fees from the beginning, and know or are willing to determine whether health insurance will cover the costs. Good health practitioners patiently answer all the patient's questions, including those concerning the practitioner's qualifications and education. They never promise a complete or immediate cure, are not on principle opposed to conventional or alternative medicine, and don't object if the patient wants to get a second opinion.

Sources for Products

Frontier Natural Products
PO Box 299
Norway, IA 52318
phone: (319) 227-7996
fax: (319) 227-7966
www.frontiercoop.com
The products distributed include natural remedies, Rosemary Gladstar, and herbal supplements.

Gritman Corporation
PO Box 2009
Friendswood, TX 77549-2009
phone: (888) 474-8626
fax: (281) 996-0138
mall6.register.com/gritman
Black Cumin and many other spices and herbs are available through Gritman's on-line catalog. Consumers may also purchase essential oil blends, home care products, stones, and books and publications.

Herbs Depot, LLC
205 Willow Way
Gatlinburg, TN 37738
fax: (423) 430-7257
http://herbs-depot.com
Herb Depot distributes herbs, oils, spices, and teas.

HerbalBath.com
15602 Olde Highway 80
Flinn Springs, CA 92021
phone: (619) 390-3525
fax: (619) 390-7148
www.herbalbath.com
Natural herbal bath products are available on-line.

Herbal Elements
6800 SW 40 St #655
Miami, FL 33155
fax: (305) 669-6702
http://www.herbalelements.com/english/buy.htm
Supplier of herbal extracts.

Kneipp Corporation of America
105-107 Stonehurst Court
Northvale, NJ 07647
phone: (800) 937-4372 or (201) 750-0600)
Kneipp products are available through this source.

Kombucha Magic Mushroom Farms, Inc.
PO Box 20717 Cherokee Station
New York, NY 10021-0074
phone: (212) 249-4463
www.kombucha.net/product.html
A primary source for kombucha culture.

Kombucha Manna International
Beverley B. Ferguson
2 Alexander Lane
Croton-on-Hudson, NY 10520
www.bestweb.net/-om-kmi/
KMI specializes in Kombucha Manna Drops, a pure extract of KMI Organic Kombucha Colinies.

Lifewayfoods
6431 W. Oakton
Morton Grove, IL 60053
phone: (847) 967-1010
fax: (847) 967-6558
http://kefir.com
Lifeway's product lines are devoted to speciality dairy foods for health-conscious consumers (Kefir).

Lotus Herbs & Holistic Health Institute
4245 Capitola Road, Suite 103
Capitola, CA 95010
phone: (831) 479-1667 or (800) 815-6887
fax: (831) 479-1951
www.lotusayurveda.com
Consumers can browse the large selection of lotus herbs and herbal remedies on-line. The Holistic Health Institute provides information on Ayureveda, diet and lifestyle, products and treatments, pancha karma, and rejuvenation and detoxification therapy.

Miller Rexall Drugs Inc.
87 Broad Street
Atlanta, GA 30303
phone: (800) 863-5654
www.mindspring.com
A large selection of herbs are available through mail-order, including European Mistletoe.

Red Mountain Remedies
6350 N. Valley View Road
Tucson, AZ 85718
phone: (888) 791-8333
fax: (520) 299-8333
redmtremedies.com
This Arizona-based company's product line includes natural remedies for common ailments—Chinese herbs, Western herbs, and homeopathic remedies.

Viable Herbal Solutions
P.O. Box 969
Morrisville, PA 19067-0969
phone: (800) 505-9475
fax: (800) 505-9476
http://www.viable-herbal.com
Supplies herbal health products.

Organizations:

American Botanical Council
PO Box 144345
Austin, TX 78714-4345
phone: (512) 926-4900
fax: (512) 926-2345
www.herbalgram.org
Provides information concerning the medicinal use of herbs and plants.

Herb Research Foundation
1007 Pearl Street, Suite 200
Boulder, CO 80302
phone: (303) 449-2265
fax: (303) 449-7849
www.herbs.org
Provides information concerning the medicinal use of herbs and plants.

The Herb Society of America
9019 Kirtland Chardon Road
Kirtland, Ohio 44094
phone: (440) 256-0514
fax: (440) 256-0541
http://www.herbsociety.org
Provides information concerning the use of herbs.

Resource Directory

For Further Reading

Breedlove Garber, Greta. *Herbal Home Spa: Naturally Refreshing Wraps, Rubs, Lotions, Masks, Oils, and Scrubs.* Pownal: Storey Books, 1998.

Britton, Jade, and Tamara Kircher. *The Complete Book of Home Herbal Remedies: A Holistic Guide to Understanding and Treating Common Ailments with Herbs.* Willowdale: Firefly Books, 1998.

Chevallier, Andrew. *Encyclopedia of Medicinal Plants.* New York: DK Publishing, 1996.

Dincin, Dian. *Ancient Healing Secrets: Practical Herbal Remedies from Around the World That Work Today.* Tonawanda: Crescent Books, 1997.

Editors of Time Life Books. *The Alternative Advisor: The Complete Guide to Natural Therapies and Alternative Treatments.* New York: Time Life, 1997.

Elias, Jason, and Shelagh Ryan Masline. *A–Z Guide to Healing Herbal Remedies.* New York: Dell Publishing Company, 1995.

Hoffman, David. *The Complete Illustrated Holistic Herbal: A Safe and Practical Guide to Making and Using Herbal Remedies.* Rockport: Elements, 1996.

Kavasch, E. Barrie. *American Indian Healing Arts: Herbs, Rituals, and Remedies for Every Season of Life.* New York: Bantam Doubleday Dell Publishers, 1999.

Lad, Vasant. *The Complete Book of Ayurvedic Home Remedies.* New York: Harmony Books, 1998.

McGuffin, Michael. *American Herbal Products Association's Botanical Safety Handbook.* Boca Raton: CRC Press, 1997.

Ody, Penelope. *Complete Medicinal Herbal.* New York: DK Publishing, 1993.

Pahlow, Mannfried. *Healing Plants.* Hauppauge, New York: Barron's Educational Series, Inc., 1993.

Peirce, Andrea, John A. Gans, and Andrew T. Weil. *American Pharmaceutical Association Practical Guide to Natural Medicines.* New York: William Morrow & Company, 1999.

Selby, Anna. *Ancient and Healing Art of Chinese Herbalism.* Berkeley: Ulysses Press, 1998.

Shealy, Norman. *The Illustrated Encyclopedia of Healing Remedies.* Rockport: Elements, 1999.

Thiess, Barbara, and Peter Thiess. *The Family Herbal: A Guide to Natural Health Care for Yourself and Your Children from Europe's Leading Herbalist.* Rochester: Healing Arts Press, 1993.

Thomas, Lalitha. *10 Essential Herbs: Everybody's Handbook to Health.* Prescott: Hohm Press, 1995.

Tyler, Varro, E., and Steven Foster. *Tyler's Honest Herbal: A Sensible Guide to the Use of Herbs and Related Remedies.* Binghamton: Haworth Press.

Vukovis, Laurel. *14-Day Herbal Cleansing.* Princeton: Prentice Hall, 1997.

White, Linda B., and Sunny Mavor. *Kids, Herbs, and Health: A Parent's Guide to Natural Remedies.* Chicago: Independent Publisher's Group, 1999.

Index

Index

Credits

About the Author

Tanja Hirschsteiner is a freelance medical journalist who lives in Munich. After completing her studies in Romance languages and psychology, she earned her degree as a licensed Healing Practitioner. She has been studying and researching alternative as well as conventional medical therapies and treatments for many years.

Photo Credits

Bavaria/Stock Imagery: page 152
Sigurd Doeppel: Front cover, pages 6, 8, 14, 76, 82, 89, 102, 112, 120, 150, 180
Hermann Eisenbeiss: pages 7, 115, 126, 144, back cover, top
Manfred Jahreiss: page 63
Gudrun Kaiser: page 26
Ulla Kimmig: pages 160, 161, 164
Susanne Kracke: page 67
Michael Leis: Back cover, middle
Mauritius-AGE: page 46
Manfred Pforr: pages 9, 95, 96, 99, 118, 128, 145
Reinhard-Animal Photography: pages 2, 3, 4, 5, 6, 7, 24, 29, 31, 43, 55, 56, 60, 77, 79, 90, 92, 99, 100, 106, 109, 121, 123, 130, 134, 137, 138, 140, 147
Thomas von Salomon: page 167, back cover, bottom
Reiner Schmitz: pages 4, 7, 12, 17, 20, 23, 33, 38, 59, 85, 104, 125, 151, 155, 157, 162
Stock Food: page 74
Toni Stone: pages 133, 143
Studio Teubner: pages 14, 25, 37, 41, 49, 68, 73

Published originally under the title: *Von Apfelessig bis Weißdorn Die besten Haus-und Naturheilmittel*
Copyright © 1998 by Grafe und Unzer Verlag GmbH. Munchen
English translation copyright © 2000 by Barron's Educational Series, Inc., Hauppauge, New York
English translation by Irene Rosko-Lustenberger

All inquiries should be addressed to:
Barron's Educational Series, Inc.
250 Wireless Boulevard
Hauppauge, New York 11788
http://www.barronseduc.com

Library of Congress Catalog Card No. 99-62849
International Standard Book No. 0-7641-1220-1

Printed in Hong Kong
9 8 7 6 5 4 3 2

Important Note
This manual contains advice on how to treat ailments with tried-and-true home and natural remedies. It is up to the reader to accept the responsibility of determining whether, and to what extent, he or she chooses to use natural remedies for treating his or her ailments. Please read and pay attention to the warnings in the text, as well as to the information regarding the limitations to self-treatment on page 13. Follow the instructions regarding dosage and proper use. If you are under the care of a physician, please inform him or her of your intention to treat yourself with home or natural remedies.